The Ideology of Community Care

THE IDEOLOGY OF
COMMUNITY
CARE

DAVID SKIDMORE

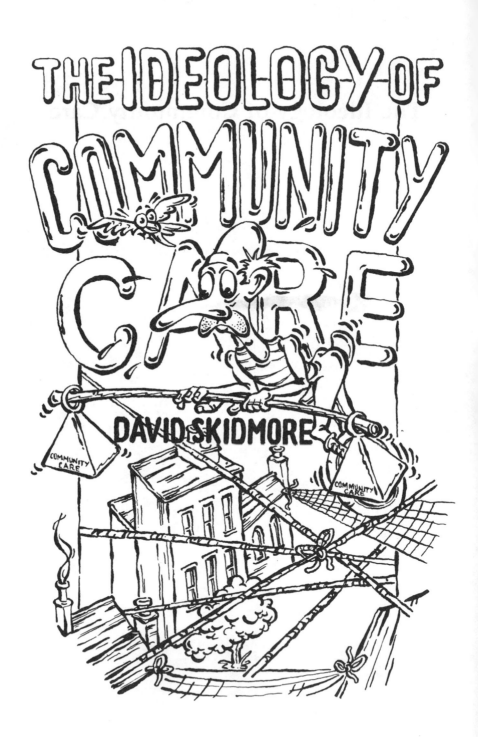

Original artwork courtesy of Paul D. Folland (Diablo)

The Ideology of Community Care

David Skidmore

Head of Department, Department of Health Care Studies
The Manchester Metropolitan University, UK

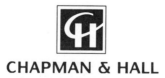

CHAPMAN & HALL

London · Glasgow · Weinheim · New York · Tokyo · Melbourne · Madras

Published by Chapman & Hall, 2–6 Boundary Row, London SE1 8HN, UK

Chapman & Hall, 2–6 Boundary Row, London SE1 8HN, UK

Blackie Academic & Professional, Wester Cleddens Road, Bishopbriggs, Glasgow G64 2NZ, UK

Chapman & Hall GmbH, Pappelallee 3, 69469 Weinheim, Germany

Chapman & Hall USA, One Penn Plaza, 41st Floor, New York NY 10119, USA

Chapman & Hall Japan, ITP-Japan, Kyowa Building, 3F, 2–2–1 Hirakawacho, Chiyoda-ku, Tokyo 102, Japan

Chapman & Hall Australia, Thomas Nelson Australia, 102 Dodds Street, South Melbourne, Victoria 3205, Australia

Chapman & Hall India, R. Seshadri, 32 Second Main Road, CIT East, Madras 600 035, India

Distributed in the USA and Canada by Singular Publishing Group Inc., 4284 41st Street, San Diego, California 92105

First edition 1994

© 1994 David Skidmore

Phototypeset in Palatino 10/12pt by Intype, London
Printed in Great Britain by St Edmundsbury Press, Bury St Edmunds, Suffolk

ISBN 0 412 47740 8   1 56593 145 9 (USA)

A catalogue record for this book is available from the British Library

Library of Congress Catalog Card Number: 9472014

♾ Printed on permanent acid-free text paper, manufactured in accordance with ANSI/NISO Z39.48–1992 AND ANSI/NISO Z39.48–1984 (Permanence of Paper).

This book is dedicated with loving memories of:

Marjorie Skidmore
Mable Dixon
Percy Copley

When the lights of your lives were extinguished
A corner in the rooms of our lives
Became forever dark.

Contents

Acknowledgements

No work is truly original and this text owes acknowledgement to those people who have helped shaped my thinking and stimulated my thoughts over several years. In reality these people are far too numerous to mention by name, but the following deserve special mention: Professor Joel Richman, Professor Ronald Frankenberg, Ray Jobling, Alan Davis and John Brown for academic stimulation; Fred Raphael, James Mitchell, Julian Mitchell and Iris Murdoch for provoking thought; Walter Skidmore for being contentious, argumentative and generally eccentrically sane.

Introduction

In this text I hope to develop an ideology of community care. It is my contention that community care has become a background expectancy in recent years. A background expectancy is something that we all appear to agree a common meaning and accept that it exists without any evidence other than personal belief. Friendship, love and caring are similar expectancies (Skidmore, 1986). There is a tendency to invest belief in the existence of these relationships without the empirical evidence to support their existences. In many ways it is the simple acceptance of feelings; a feeling that such things should exist to emphasize our humanity. Skidmore (1986) argues that people subscribe to such beliefs in order to give anchorage to their own worth within the world. The value of this anchorage is reinforced by the romantic aspect within fiction; consequently, because of television, a consensus of agreement regarding the meaning of background expectancies is shared by large groups of people.

Community care can be added to this list since it is increasingly becoming romanticized as a concept. Community care is the answer to client-centred care, it is often mooted (HMSO, 1988); even though many clients are not consulted about such care (Torrey, 1985). On face value community care appears to be the product of the 'professionals'; what they feel is best for the client. This places the professional firmly in a parental role and the client in the role of child – a relationship antagonistic to the ethos of community care. Attempts to stimulate thought regarding an ideology may, at least, promote dialogue between the many community carers, even if only to debunk this text.

An ideology is defined (*Oxford English Dictionary*) as:
... a science of ideas; visionary speculation ...

I'm not convinced that one can gather a science of ideas since ideas are personal to many people and, consequently, quite diverse. Additionally, science is based on understanding. It suggests that which has been observed, empirically, and that such events can subsequently be repeated and measured. This, in turn, provides a body of knowledge, a framework of 'normality' against which other events can be compared (or measured). There would be, then, a definition of 'normal' community upon which all 'normal' communities would be based.

Back to the definition of ideology. I tend to favour the latter definition providing one removes the visionary. An ideology of community care, in my sense, is speculation about a collection of ideas about care in the community and those themes that are supportive and/or antagonistic of both care and community.

Community care has attracted much comment and explanation over several years (McKeown and Lowe, 1976; Carr *et al.*, 1980; Glendenning, 1982; Butterworth and Skidmore, 1983; Skidmore and Friend, 1984; Brooker and Simmonds, 1986; Orr, 1986). There is a difference of opinion between the pundits on the very meaning of the term. Is it care by the community? Care in the community? Whichever option one chooses includes assumptions:

1. that there is a community;
2. that the community cares;
3. that formal structures (such as hospitals) can be separated from the community;
4. that communities are safe and friendly places.

These assumptions create an even larger assumption that **communities are static**. Communities are there because they have always been . . . and because they used to care they still do.

Some historians argue that communities are a modern, idealistic creation. People did not interact on a regular basis and met only to trade which was a poor medium for the growth of community (Mitchell, 1986). That was then and this is now. Communities exist because we have created them. They exist because we (the professionals and the people) want them to . . . we have our own ideas about them and our experience of it. In addition we have gathered perceptions of the experiences of others (our parents, peers and pundits). Community exists today in the same sense that a country exists: a person can live in his country knowing he belongs to a network and is understood and understands others. The person being cared for in the community will be seen in varying degrees of 'alien-ness', as though visiting a foreign country:

> Being in a foreign country means walking a tightrope high above the ground without the net afforded a person by the country where he has a family, colleagues and friends, and where he can easily say what he has to say in a language he has known from childhood . . .
>   (Kundera, 1984)

This text will utilize the leitmotif of geographical terms and families in order to develop a meaning to community. The community is viewed as a country, the natives are those families that make up the community and we shall examine the emigres, visitors, exiles and refugees.

Above all I do not offer this as a definitive text, it is purely seminal. Nor is it intended to be a guidebook or a manual of thought. The text is based on empirical study, literature, philosophical diatribe and experience and as such becomes a work of pure speculation intended to prompt discussion. I have tried to steer clear of jargon, although it will inevitably creep in liberally. If this book stimulates thought and debate about how we treat others, be that in the community or within the institution, then it has succeeded.

Finally this book addresses the whole arena of community care since it targets people and not categories.

REFERENCES

Brooker, C. and Simmonds, S. (1986) *Community Psychiatric Nursing: a social perspective*, Heinemann, London.

Butterworth, C.A. and Skidmore, D. (1983) *Caring for the Mentally Ill in the Community*, Croom Helm, London.

Carr, P.J., Butterworth, C.A. and Hodges, B.E. (1980) *Community Psychiatric Nursing*, Churchill Livingstone, Edinburgh.

Glendenning, F. (ed.) (1982) *Care in the Community*, Department of Adult Education, University of Keele.

HMSO (1988) *Community Care – Agenda for Action* (Griffiths Report). HMSO, London.

Kundera, M. (1984) *The Unbearable Lightness of Being*, Faber and Faber, London.

McKeown, T. and Lowe, C.R. (1974) *An Introduction to Social Medicine*, Blackwell, Oxford.

Mitchell, J. (1986) Interview in The sociology of friendship, (ed. D. Skidmore), University of Keele, unpublished PhD Thesis.

Orr, J. (ed.) (1986) *Women's Health in the Community*, Wiley, London.

Skidmore, D. (1986) The sociology of friendship: historical, literary and empirical perspectives. University of Keele, unpublished PhD thesis.

Skidmore, D. and Friend, W. (1984) The effectiveness of community psychiatric nursing. The Manchester Metropolitan University, unpublished research report.

Torrey, E.F. (1985) *Surviving Schizophrenia*. Harper and Row, London.

David Skidmore
Manchester, 1994

Community

An exploration of meanings and images
of community

CHAPTER 1

The geography of being

Most texts of this nature attempt, at some time or other, to offer a definition of community (Carr, Butterworth and Hodges, 1980; Brooker and Simmonds, 1989). This text will make no such attempt since, in terms of a person-centred approach, it is irrelevant. If a person feels that he belongs in a particular location then that is his community. A therapist will not help him more by having a mechanistic understanding of what community should be. Frankenberg (1975) argues that each person sees himself as the centre of his social network and, one would suggest, his community. The therapist should, then, make attempts to discover what community means to a person.

This text takes, as a framework, a geographical context. It is concerned with location in its broadest sense. A person may feel located within a particular place, within a certain group and within a certain structure. His life may develop its own atlas where he will recognize boundaries, contours, safe lands and rough seas that will help him to plan his journey through life. This atlas will help him make predictions and develop expectations about his 'globe'. When we think of our world we do not conjure images of land and sea; we think also of climate, vegetation, different people, different cultures and different governments. Similarly a person's globe conjures multiple images. Like the world he is more than a superficial image. He has a biology (structure), a sociology (culture), a psychology (people) and a political (government) dimension (Hodges, 1986).

Concentrating on the theme of physical location for the moment, the world is broken down into land and sea. The land into countries, countries into cities, towns and villages (habitation) and the rural. The inhabited areas are further broken down into specific areas (e.g. Bethnal Green area of London). A person's physical location is similar. He will find himself located in a specific area, initially through no choice of his own; he may have been born and brought up in Bethnal Green. This aspect of his location will have an institutionalized aspect in that it existed prior to his birth, may well exist after his death, will have an existence and history separate from him (Bilton et al., 1987). This offers a meaningful structure to his life, a backdrop against which he can test and try his personal development. This backdrop becomes part of his personal country and his community.

If we were to picture a person's community as his country, to some extent that is from where he draws an identity. He becomes located, i.e. English, American or French. He has the use of a language that is understood by those who share his community. He has a safety net of relationships (family, colleagues and friends) that he believes will cushion him when he falls from this location. He knows which part of this country is safe, which is unsafe and which areas are unknown. In short he will have clear expectations, based upon experience, of how others will react to him in any given encounter. He has grown with his community and the people around him, familiar and not so familiar, have grown with him. Consequently, he has such familiarity with his 'community' that it causes no concern if he were to leave it for a while, for a holiday. It is perfectly normal to take 'a break'. One can look forward to an adventure 'abroad' in the knowledge that the safety net of one's community is easily within reach. Often we test that net by climbing higher and higher. Using the geographical example a person may start testing his net by visiting those parts of his country about which he knows nothing. The child may inch his way to the bottom of the street and, in time, turn the corner. Over time this seems incredibly familiar and he yearns for new streets until he 'knows' his local geography. This prompts him to visit new locations, new towns and cities. His culture is geared to this in the form of the annual holiday when parents structure a visit to new places. When the child becomes adult he continues the tradition of discovery and may seek the ultimate adventure of exploring abroad.

Visiting a strange country is often a pleasurable experience. The visit is often the product of a reasonably informed choice, a holiday for example. We can prepare for such a journey with various guides and maps that are available. The tourist is often experienced in 'home travel' and has developed the sense of security that 'home' is always waiting. Home (and community) is that place which offers succour against the stresses and strains of everyday life ... a haven. This helps the person plan sojourns to new places. When you are involved in the decision to visit you know where you are coming from and where you are intending to go to, and more importantly where you intend to return to. Without this information maps are pretty useless.

When you arrive in the country you have chosen to visit you will have some idea of the arena, e.g. that a different language is spoken; this information may stimulate you to obtain a phrase book. You may also have spoken to previous visitors who might have given you details of where to visit and where to avoid. In short you will have carried out some research that will help you to develop landmarks to navigate the new country.

Imagine that you woke up one morning not knowing where you were or how you got there. You find yourself in a place where the natives speak a similar language but seem to have different meanings. Since you have no idea where you are you cannot buy a map and similarly cannot locate the language that would enable you to buy a phrasebook to give you the wherewithal to ask where you are. Kundera (1984) puts this rather succinctly:

> Being in a foreign country means walking a tightrope high above the ground without the net afforded a person by the country where he has a family, colleagues and friends, and where he can easily say what he has to say in a language he has known from childhood ...

Being in one's own country offers security. It is far more than having access to a familiar language, one is connected and has an identity that is mutually recognized by the 'community'. Consider what is meant by 'identity'. You know who you are and so do people that you know. To some extent those people with whom you are connected will have some knowledge of your history. They will be able to explain that you are: '... so and so's son/daughter'. Consequently 'identity' has two parameters: personhood and personship. Personhood is that inner concept, who we believe we are; personship is the recognition by others that we are who we claim to be.

Personhood offers the individual the opportunity to order his life with reference to others. I am a friend, husband, father, brother or some noun that is recognized. In other words he takes his identity from what is perceived to be previously defined roles. Expectations exist about these roles and a prime expectation is that others have an understanding of what such roles mean; they can locate them within a framework of meaning. The framework of meaning, in this sense, allows us to construct a series of networks, since a role cannot exist in isolation; i.e. without others to relate to any role becomes meaningless. One cannot be a brother without one's brother, or a father without children. Hence a person's first network is that of kinship. Within the network we have a location and a sense of identity. The feeling of belonging will develop for those who are kept within the network and feelings of rejection for those who are excluded or marginalized. This network has become accepted as a norm by society to such an extent that those who display deviant behaviour are often thought to come from a faulty network (broken home or poor family ties).

Norms are those aspects of societal life that we understand everyone else accepts as the right way of life. To a large extent these are inherited and possess history: i.e. they were norms before we were born and we are schooled in them from an early age. Nietzsche (1977) would argue that these are merely the reflections of the ideals of a society's greatest man. In other words a powerful person or group of persons enforce their beliefs onto the rest of us. In many societies there will exist a written code on which these are based, usually intertwined with religion (e.g. the ten commandments). Nietzsche's premise is that we are individuals and consequently function chaotically; onto this chaos an unnatural order has been enforced and this is supported by myth.

Every society has a body of myth: the Greek legends, Arthurian legends and many more. Such legends tend to extol the finer qualities of humanity: courage, love and justice. In many ways they are moralistic and reinforce the notion that society is more important than the person. In Arthurian legend Lancelot woos and wins his best friend's girl, Guinevere, and the result is war and the end of the then known civilized society. The moral is that not only should you not commit adultery but also do not betray a friend since the retribution far outweighs the original sin.

It could be argued that similar myths exist about society. We are schooled into accepting a notion of family, love, friendship and several other qualities.

During the late fifties the media warned of the fragmentation of the extended family. Many social scientists warned of the subsequent consequences: crime, delinquency and a slip in the quality of life. However, it has been suggested that the extended family is a modern myth. Mitchell (1986) suggests that the extended family only came about by way of the industrial revolution. People started living longer because they had the wherewithal to buy food rather than live from the land. They moved to towns where work was on offer and generations of the same family developed networks of mutual help and support. However, by the mid 1950s the rise of the affluent worker occurred (Lockwood, 1958). The new affluence gave the worker the opportunity to move from his place of birth and purchase a means of transport that allowed him to commute to work. A consequence of geographical mobility meant the erosion of the supposed extended family and the dominance of the 'so-called' nuclear family. In recent times we have heard similar warnings concerning the demise of the nuclear family.

The family will be examined later, but for now let us consider whether or not the community is merely a collection of families and similar networks. The safest thing that we can say about communities is that they contain people. Again, a definition is not really useful, a meaning, however, is a different matter. For those who have strong family ties the community may merely be a location for his/her family. Others may have weak family ties and strong friendship links. The concept of neighbours is another aspect that may signify community to some people. In reality these are the anchors that a person uses to construct his/her community reality. Several sociologists and social psychologists have suggested that if a person were to attempt to write down the names of everyone that he/

she knows then the list would never be completed. You may care to try this on a long train ride.

Families, friends, acquaintances, neighbours and lovers are nouns that provide each person with a geography of being, i.e. a sense of location. We hold the expectation that they mean the same to others that we interact with. Skidmore (1986) suggests that these are merely background expectancies; points of social consensus of meaning that may radically differ between persons. When investigating friendship Skidmore (1986) discovered that many subjects were describing themself when they described friends and that friends offered opposing views of their description. Furthermore, the concept of friendship was offered meaning by way of actions that would never be tested:

> This person is a close friend because if I were ever to need money I could ask this person and they would give me money ... I never would but I know that I could.

There may be security in this feeling that there is a depth to relationships. There is no evidence that love exists other than what is read and what others declare; but generally most people accept that love in some form exists. There is, however, a sense of predictability in accepting the existence of love and friendship. To feel loved and befriended offers meaning, worth and acceptance to one's life; one is worthy because others like one.

In similar ways we attribute meaning to life in other ways: by playing and recognizing roles. Not only does this help a person to locate others within a geography of being, it also allows others to locate the person. Buber (1970) suggests that we can only ever gain a perception of another's experience, we can never share that experience. Therefore each person's experience of the world is unique and, consequently, each person constructs different meanings about things. We are, however, able to understand the sense of each others meaning by the way in which society is constructed. There are norms, social mores and formal rules that are relatively fixed and which everyone learns. There are mechanisms in place that will deal with those persons who choose to ignore or break the rules. This structure allows people to make predictions about everyday life (Homans, 1951). It indicates how a person should behave in any given situation (Marris, 1974). A diagrammatic representation of the 'conservative impulse' is useful at this stage, and is given in Figure 1.1.

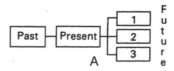

Figure 1.1 The conservative impulse.

When a person encounters any event at A (Figure 1.1), he looks back into his past in order to review any data collected that will give clues about how to deal with the event. At the same time he looks around in the present to gather clues from his environment about the best way to behave in this event. He then conjectures behaviours and acts on one, which immediately is filed into the past for future reference (judged on success/failure). Given a lifetime of this behaviour quite extensive data banks can be developed as a source of reference. Perhaps this is why we appear to gain more confidence in social situations as we grow older (and more experienced).

Let us break this down a little further.

PAST

The computations of a person's past are probably infinite. To begin with he or she has no control over the location he or she is born into. The relevant genes will dictate sex, appearance and these, in turn, society's reaction towards him or her. The geographical location will dictate, to some extent, the living conditions, type of school, peer group and life chances that one is exposed to. Indeed this 'past' will contrive to locate the person securely in the present: verbal skill, occupation, wealth, marriage partner and peers. To paraphrase Burke (1978), where a person is now depends on where he or she has come from. The personal location can vary significantly; the child may have both loving parents, a single parent or be orphaned. Each computation will carry a specific stigma. On a simplistic level, the geography of being can be viewed as the history of a person's society.

At this level it could be argued that a child (for the sake of simplicity male, although no sexism is implied) is born into a predetermined backdrop, rich with meaning, rules and codes. A large portion of the child's reality is blueprinted by the macro-society (i.e. British). The colours that enrich the blueprint are selected by the micro-society (the subculture of the town) and over time the development of personhood may influence the shade of the colour. The shade of the colour will depend on the result of interplay between him and his 'community'. His history will paint him as having high or low status, breeding or vulgarity, normality or madness. How he is viewed (painted) is his backdrop and that backdrop will shape his own expectancies, as it did for his parents and peers. To some extent it determines the approach he takes with him to any encounter. He is located within his history which has been shaped by his 'society's' greatest men – back to Nietzsche again. To a large extent, those things that he has embraced from his history are myths in true Nietzscherian style. Order has been forced onto chaos; he constructs meaning from his random encounters with people by categorizing them:

friend, family or lover. When he displays the appropriate behaviour and the other party reciprocates then the myth becomes reality until the act wears thin. Lovers who proclaimed love at first sight are quick to explain, on separation, that it was not love after all ... merely infatuation. Ideals are protected from real scrutiny for fear that they will be exposed as myth.

Society, then, provides a person with a structure with which he can approach encounters, a vocabulary of interaction that is shared with other natives, but only he, as a person, can ascribe meaning to any event. His experience of his reality is unique (Buber, 1970). In a philosophical sense his journey through life is quite lonely. He will, of course, be conditioned to certain needs by the structure he has learned to recognize, the structure that is society's gift (Maslow, 1968). He will feel a need to be accepted, to be recognized and to have relationships. These are needs inherited from his past and the past that existed before he did; they are part of the structure developed to give order and predictability to chaos. The person's past is all those events that occurred before the 'now' from his year zero. All that data collected by observation and overheard from parents and peers; formal conditioning absorbed from the media

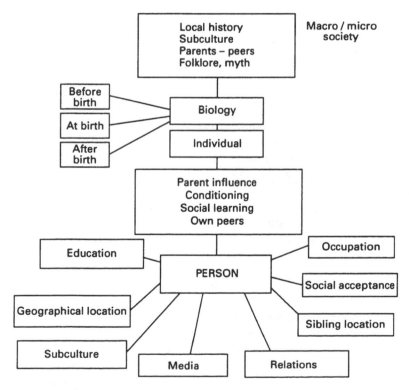

Figure 1.2 'Personship'.

(fact and fiction); those experiences endured because of his geography of being. In short a person is the product of biology, sociology, psychology, history and politics. We could graphically represent this, as shown in Figure 1.2.

Not only is this a model of a person's past it is very much his present since all the influences possess fluidity in that they change and exert more or less influence over time. You will note that the diagram refers to both the individual and the person. Schutz (1962) suggests that we are born individuals but from the moment we interact with society we become persons (the social actor). One would add to this that we carry both persona with us in everyday encounters: a public and a private self.

THE PRESENT

The past impinges on the present so much that it is difficult to separate them. The here and now rapidly slips into the recent past and, to some degree, enables the person to rationalize actions after the event, even though they may have been initiated irrationally. It has been suggested, above, that we are born into a structured backdrop that we will call our community and/or society. Values devised in our past constantly impinge on the present. We learn to function on several agendas. For example, most people accept that lying is wrong and yet will encourage children to lie; we generate the social lie . . . or tact. This is because there is a basic script for interaction, a code of what is right and proper. The present cannot exist without reference to the past, because each situation is charged with expectation . . . a notion of what the future outcome is likely to be, in turn deducted from cues picked up in the present. Nietzsche (1977) argues that without history there is no society and that society is the product of myth, folklore and history. History provides meaning to the here and now, consequently, without a past there can be no present and no geography of being. The past provides a point of reference which offers meaning to the present. The blurring of past, present and future can best be seen through role.

ROLE

Nietzsche's (1977) suggestion that order is forced onto chaos may have its illustration through roles. Roles aid a person in the application of the conservative impulse through everyday life. They help to construct, maintain and give meaning to reality. Consider the role of parent: there are no formal classes that instruct a person on how to be a parent and yet most people have a notion of how parents should behave. Much of the expectations we have about roles are acquired from the society we are born into; that is they are the product of history. In order to negotiate a path through everyday life most people have many roles, such as female, sister, mother, employee, daughter, teacher, wife and friend. Each role will demand different behavioural displays, each display having a historical component which is built upon from past knowledge, modified by present experience, shaped by future expectations and filed away as data for future reference.

Let us consider the role of male. Although there is no recognizable formal classes in maleness there does exist a 'role-script'. This is firmly located within a person's social location: the perceived actions of other males, those behaviours which parents encourage and discourage; how the male is portrayed through the media. All these will help develop a 'normal' view of males which a male person will try to mirror. Buber (1970) argues that we respond to our perception of others, we can never experience their experiences; therefore our perception becomes synonymous with their experience, i.e. they become what we see. There will be differences in role displays in public and those in private since public displays are far more formalized (Goffman, 1969) and this difference will be explored in the next chapter.

Role display is more than a simple expression of 'self'. A person's self is complex, it has learned to work with several agendas: public and private roles are two variables. Added to the public and private display (private is the display revealed to intimate relations) is the inner and outer self. Most social psychologists and sociologists refer to the outer self when reporting human behaviour. The inner self refers to those parts of a person that only they know. Raphael (1976) offers a succinct explanation with:

> They asked him how he had managed for so long to lead a double life. He replied that nothing was easier. As long as he could keep just one chamber of his castle locked and its contents safe from scrutiny, Bluebeard was model husband, reliable father and responsible citizen.
>
> (Raphael, 1976)

Ellis (1991) takes this notion of the secret chamber further in his portrayal of the serial killer. Bateman (Ellis's character) keeps his two lives apart: the public self (outer) of the successful yuppie where encounters are almost scripted, and the private (inner) killer who breaks the rules. Periodically Bateman tries to enforce his inner self onto the mechanistic outside world but it is contained by others who treat his outbursts as a joke or a result of drink. Ellis (1991) makes it perfectly clear that when another person asks how you are they don't really want to know, they are merely playing the social game. In the Dostoyevsky (1966) tradition Bateman is similar to Raskolnikov after inflicting his secret chamber onto the outer world: both start to fragment as people and lose control. Raskolnikov's argument is that there is nothing wrong with murdering an old, female money lender who most people hate if a larger number of people benefit from the death. Problems arise when he tries to make sense of his actions after the event: his action is the past, the present is not related to his secret action and yet he is used to functioning on that basis. Hence he translates all actions in reference to his action and becomes convinced that the policeman knows he is guilty. His subsequent behaviour is based on that of the guilty suspect and his crime is discovered. Ellis (1991) does not offer a logical outcome to Bateman's life, we are left experiencing Bateman's disintegrating personality after he has allowed inner and outer selves to mix.

In short, society has mechanisms to contain attempts to enforce individual beliefs upon society. We have a consensus of what is normal and anyone stepping outside that norm is abnormal. To reveal inner self is an abnormal act because it does not concur with the majority view. Social life is relatively ordered and predictable. We ask someone how they are because it is the done thing. If they start to tell us how they are then they are not responding as expected and border on the abnormal. The outer self helps to maintain the predictability and, in turn, is maintained by timetables.

The geography of being, that is a person's reality, is punctuated by points of progression. Day becomes night; day consists of morning, afternoon and evening; it is further categorized by mealtimes . . . all offering a notion of progression and predictability. Days add up to weeks, which add up to months which become years. We flower the year with special days that indicate certain behaviours: Christmas when we should love our fellow men, or as Lehrer (1968) puts it:

On Christmas day you can't get sore
Your fellow man you must adore
You've time to hate him all the more
The other three hundred and sixty-four.

In order to add greater predictability we ascribe certain signs to categories of the year which we refer to as birth signs; people born under these signs supposedly inherit certain characteristics . . . again offering predictability. Under this scheme people become typical Taurians or perfect Piscians and even arrogant Ariens. An example of forcing order onto chaos?

A person's life is similarly timetabled: he has a period as a baby, child, youth, adult, old person. There are classical ages where certain things are expected: periods of childhood development, adolescence . . . where specific behaviours are anticipated. For example, although you will know that entering into a sexual act is okay from 16 years, you cannot vote or drink until you are 18.

FUTURE

Whilst we may think that some aspects of our society are ridiculous they have a purpose: they ensure the existence of a common future . . . something we can expect, anticipate and realize. Without an ordered past and present the future would be chaotic. Chaos would be a threat to society because it would inhibit interaction. With order we can expect, with reasonable accuracy, how a person will react in any given situation . . . without it we are lost. The FBI have tried to enforce order onto the character profiles of serial killers with little success in detection rates (Wilson and Seaman, 1992). Most authorities agree that serial killers are successful because of the randomness of their activities . . . that is that it lacks order.

In reality one could argue that the future is a myth. It only exists because we will it to exist. The future may well be a consequence of that which we have engineered because of our expectations. Lippman (1922) suggests that we define first and then see; in other words we see that which we wish to see. If this is so we may well select those actions that reinforce our preconceived ideas, as in confirming birth sign behaviour; or in gaining a perception of another's experience. We can stimulate a certain kind of behaviour in another person by the way we react to that person. The consequence of this activity is an extension of the present rather than a recognition of the future. Most people know what they will be doing tomorrow with reasonable certainty. This expectation is based on what was done today and on personal history. Hence we can argue that the present is an extension of the past. If this is so then the future is also an extension of the past.

In a totally mechanistic world this would be true. Asimov (1962) exemplified this in his 'Foundation' novels with the concept of psychohistory: that the future could be predicted by study of the past. What such a theory ignores is the chaotic nature of the future. The future does not obey rules and may deviate from the predicted path. When attempts to contain it by alternative classifications fail we enter a period of normlessness or anomie (Durkheim, 1970), when the conservative impulse fails to guide a person in an acceptable direction. Fortunately, for most people, society is structured in such a way as to prevent everyday anomie. The majority of roles are formalized and protected by laws, rules and tradition. The formalization of society has developed along a private to public continuum which we will explore in the next chapter. We are able to construct a view of reality by making huge chunks of life symbolic. A symbol informs; it offers far more information than its simple form. Role titles are symbolic in this sense: motherhood, lover and friend offer a great deal of information based on personal experience.

To summarize, Banks (1984) suggests that:

All our lives are symbols. Everything we do is part of a pattern we have at least some say in. The strong make their own patterns and influence other people's, the weak have their courses mapped out for them. The weak and the unlucky, and the stupid.

Banks' strong people and Nietzsche's 'obermenche' may well be those persons who feel that they have control of their lives, whilst the rest feel controlled by others, or fate, or gods. Whether we are controlled or controller depends on our skills of communicating and negotiating with the world. Caplan (1964) argues that when we are in a state of crisis we are susceptible to external control. We have already explored how crises can occur, i.e. when the conservative impulse breaks down and we enter anomie. It has been argued above that when people feel that they can make predictions about their route, i.e. their geography of being, they feel secure and in control. Knowing where you have come from helps to locate you in the here and now. As Banks (1984) puts it:

Each of us . . . may believe we have stumbled down one corridor, and that our fate is sealed and certain . . ., but a word, a glance, a slip – anything can change that, alter it entirely, and our marble hall becomes a gutter, or our rat-maze a golden path. Our destination is the same at the end, but our journey – part chosen, part determined – is different for us all, and changes even as we live and grow.

How we deal with those changes will be explored in later chapters. However, Banks is reaffirming the point made earlier that everyone's experiences of life are different. We may hide under a blanket of being Mr or Mrs Average, it helps to maintain predictability, but in reality we are all very different. When those differences manifest themselves we contain it with a new symbol. In mediaeval times if one discovered the name of the witch then one had power over her. Our logic has progressed only a short distance since those times.

In the next chapter we shall examine how we construct the wider society in order to maintain our view of reality i.e. how we project our geography of being and develop an atlas of existence.

REFERENCES

Asimov, I. (1962) *Foundation*, Panther, London.
Banks, I. (1984) *The Wasp Factory*, Futura, London.
Bilton, T., Bolton, T., Bonnett, K. et al. (1987) *Introductory Sociology*, Macmillan, London.
Brooker, C. and Simmonds, S. (1989) *Community Psychiatric Nursing: a social perspective*, Chapman and Hall, London.
Buber, M. (1970) *I and Thou*, T & T Clarke, Edinburgh.

Burke, J. (1978) *Connections*, Macmillan, London.

Carr, P.J., Butterworth, C.A. and Hodges, B.E. (1980) *Community Psychiatric Nursing*, Churchill Livingstone, Edinburgh.

Caplan, G. (1964) *Principles of Preventative Psychiatry*, Tavistock, London.

Dostoyevsky, F. (1966) *Crime and Punishment*, Penguin, Harmondsworth, Middlesex.

Durkheim, E. (1970) *Suicide: a study in sociology*, Routledge and Kegan Paul, London.

Ellis, B.E. (1991) *American Psycho*, Pan, London.

Frankenberg, R. (1975) *Communities in Britain*, Penguin, Harmondsworth, Middlesex.

Goffman, E. (1969) *The Presentation of Self in Everyday Life*, Penguin, Harmondsworth, Middlesex.

Hodges, B.E. (1986) The health career model, Unpublished, The Manchester Metropolitan University.

Homans, G.C. (1951) *The Human Group*, Routledge and Kegan Paul, London.

Kundera, M. (1984) *The Unbearable Lightness of Being*, Faber and Faber, London.

Lehrur, T. (1968) *An Evening with Tom Lehrur*, Columbia Broadcasting Systems, USA.

Lippman, W. (1922) *Public Opinion*, Macmillan, London.

Lockwood, D. (1958) *The Blackcoated Worker*, Allen and Unwin, London.

Marris, B. (1974) *Loss and Change*, Routledge and Kegan Paul, London.

Maslow, A.H. (1968) *Towards a Psychology of Being*, Van Nostrand Reinhold, New York.

Mitchell, J. (1986) Interview in The Sociology of Friendship, (D. Skidmore), University of Keele, PhD Thesis.

Nietzsche, F. (1977) *A Nietzsche Reader* (trans. R.J. Hollingdale), Penguin, Harmondsworth, Middlesex.

Raphael, F. (1976) *The Glittering Prizes*, Penguin, Harmondsworth, Middlesex.

Schutz, A. (1962) *The Problem of Social Reality: collected papers*, Martinus Nijhoff, The Hague.

Skidmore, D. (1986) The sociology of friendship: historical, literary and empirical perspectives, University of Keele, PhD Thesis.

Wilson, C. and Seaman, D. (1992) *The Serial Killers*, Virgin, London.

CHAPTER 2

The atlas of existence

An atlas is defined as a volume of maps. The term is used here to symbolize that each person's existence is composed of more than one country. A country is defined as a nation, land of birth or region. In terms of existence it is a recognizable region where the contours are familiar, the boundaries known and the culture recognized. Each country is a sphere of life, there is a social sphere, a professional sphere and an intimate sphere, each with its own language and customs. There are countries known and unknown, friendly and hostile, and each will be broken down into various states. This is our atlas. In order to give the atlas anchorage we share symbols with others which suggest that they carry the same passport. In Chapter 1 this sharing was referred to as points of social consensus; however, they could be effectively called 'constellations of agreement'. Generally, when we refer to family, we assume shared understanding. We acknowledge others as belonging to the same country and we share language and meaning with those people.

Each person's country will have states: connected areas that generally share a common identity but which are quite different. Lovers, for example, may share common friends but indulge in different dialects with each, i.e. codes of speech; one lover may reveal more to these friends than the other. Friends tend to develop special codes of speech which advertise their closeness (Skidmore, 1986). Both relationships (friends and lovers) are examples of intimacy and yet will demand different roles. Such relationships form networks that, in turn, give shape to communities. Societies are collections of people who touch each other in various ways. Relationships are never wasted because they help shape the journey through life and we cannot but help relating to others. These people that a person easily relates to are the natives of his country and help him to feel that he is located somewhere and yet our understanding of relationships is often anchored within the history of the society in which we are born. Just as a person displays an identity, so too does a collection of people; we refer to them as a collection of friends, a family or work colleagues. These titles are symbolic and infer meaning to the observer. Those onlookers who know of the title will anticipate certain behaviours from the groups. When those behaviours are witnessed (defined and then seen, Chapter 1) the onlookers feel secure and as though they belong to the same country. In this way each person recognizes landmarks common to others (constellations of agreement) which form the contours of the life map.

Each country will be an institution in its own right in that it contains history. It will have an identity separate from the person. The community is such a country. It exists in that a collection of constellations of agreement exist about it for a network of people. One could argue that it only exists because a collection of people will it to exist. The power of the individual is often discounted, but the influence of groups is well recognized (Ashe, 1955). When people get together and believe they share common meaning then for them the object of that meaning has reality. Consider the family. Many attempts have been made to reshape society by modifying the family. Experiments such as the kibbutz generally failed because persons continued to subscribe to the ideals of the family. In some cases parents secretly visited children against the rules. Children were seen as communal in that they belonged to the group and expressions of ownership negated the philosophy of the kibbutz. Whilst members agreed with the philosophy, they had problems living it once they became parents. In short it may be that the existence of the family survived because the people willed it to survive.

These 'ideals' that help construct reality become symbols of normality. These symbols of normality help a person to experience the world as an objective reality similar to our experience of the institutional world (Berger and Luckmann, 1984). People help friends and family, love parents and their children, care for siblings and so on. If a person expresses the opposite, e.g. he hates his mother, the rest of the network think him abnormal. These ideals are the 'cement' of the country, the means of binding people together in terms of neighbourliness, kinship and camaraderie. These ideals have a historical anchorage. It is not uncommon to hear people proclaim that 'people had more regard for each other in the old days'. However, one must consider that people had less chance to be other than close. There was far less geographical mobility for the majority of the population until the 1950s. The idyllic village life of pre-industrial Britain is also suspect (Mitchell, 1986). To reiterate from Chapter 1, Mitchell (1986) argues that the extended family was, in fact, a creation of the industrial revolution. People started living longer because they had the wherewithal to buy food rather than rely on the land. Consequently families tended to conglomerate in one area. The constellation of agreement was that families helped each other and this was witnessed in Young and Wilmot (1957). However, with the rise of the affluent worker (Lockwood, 1958) family members found the means to escape the family and move away, causing the sociologists of the day to pontificate about the demise of the extended family and subsequently society. However, if the extended family was artificially created within existing society it is hardly likely that its demise would destroy it; it didn't. Society as a functional system still exists.

Marriage can be described as one of the norms that is viewed by many as one of the pillars of society. Let us explore the ritual. We have arrived at a time when only one-third of marriages survive. The vows demand that one stays faithful until death parts them. In the old days, when there was little geographical mobility, it may have been relatively easy to keep such vows. Everyone knew each other and it was difficult to be private, or even believe that one could have clandestine relations. In fact, one may have made an informed choice about all the members of the opposite sex one had met and was ever likely to. The lack of geographical mobility created less opportunity for new meetings or opportunity to develop a secret life. Seen in this context it is fairly easy to understand how marriages lasted for long periods. The breakdown of marriage can be linked to the development of the 'global village'; the more people became mobile, the more people they met and the opportunity to construct a private self emerged. The 'ownership' of a private or secret life provided opportunity to develop secret relationships (Zinski and Zinski, 1973) which in turn threatened marriage. The notion of the 7-year itch was born in an attempt to explain the breakdown, or name the witch to return to the analogy in Chapter 1. As with the family, the breakdown of marriage was seen as a threat to society itself.

Accepting the family and marriage as cornerstones of society is crucial to our understanding of that which is advertised as normal. Society has developed various means to strengthen its framework and convince its members that this is right and just. Whilst most people accept that there are differences between sexes, many social scientists argue that gender differences are socially constructed (Bilton *et al.*, 1987). There is an investment in maintaining gender differences from society's point of view. A structured inequality which is generally accepted ultimately benefits the society that has produced it. Western society has strong foundations of structured inequality. A class system of some kind can be witnessed in most cultures (Bilton *et al.*, 1987). Any class system suggests that one group of people has more status than others. Within each group further classifications will exist, based on some notion of worth. The young are more valuable than the old, or men more worthy than women.

In the same way that families and marriages are important to society so too is a system of inequality. To develop such a system society requires a classification system, which we will explore later. For the moment let us examine how a person builds up his/her book of life maps which give meaning to 'community' and society.

A person is born. About that he or she has no choice, that we are aware of. Schutz (1962) argues that we are born individuals but the moment we socialize we are turned into a person. A person being a socially desirable type. What exactly is meant here? The implication is that our minds are blank and receptive to information fed in by others. To some extent this is true ... we require the maps that will guide us through life, that will help us relate to our society. The first point of socialization is with adults of some sort, whether we belong to a family or not. These adults will play a significant part in helping the individual construct a person map. The person map is a general map that has the major features but lacks the detail of the road map. To a large extent these initial features of the map will be a product of the adults' beliefs. If the adults form the person's family, that person has no reason to believe that every other person does not have a family and that his/her experiences are shared by everyone.

Humour tends to be successful because it strikes a chord of understanding in many people. Many comedians utilize their experiences of childhood to success because others recognize or have shared the experience. For example, most children who have experienced parents will remember their parent asking:

Do you want a smack?

or

I'll wipe that smile off your face in a minute.

And almost every child vows that if they ever have children they will never say those things, only to hear themselves sounding like their own parents. This is the power of that which is accepted as being normal. Traditions are passed down, mirrored and imitated. They are also reinforced.

From a fairly protected beginning we eventually sally forth and meet other persons in our community who have similarly had a basic route map etched out for them. To some extent this assists each person in confirming the basic contours of his/her embryonic atlas and, indeed, to add more detail. The person may discover that other 'families' are not exactly identical to his/her own; that there are people who are less accommodating in a social sense; people who should be avoided. Hence onwards to stereotyping.

BUILDING CONTOURS

People tend to find their way around familiar countryside by the aid of recognized features: the church, a certain hill or a bend in the road. These features make the map redundant for the native. In a similar vein 'communities' give contours to their 'existence' in order to give familiarity. The general rules of the society we are born into usually provide some contours. However, these are often reinforced by events that prompt certain behaviours. In much the same way that everyday life

builds on a timetable (Chapter 1), many 'communities' develop communal timetables that bring its members together. Not too long ago this was
a function of the church and whole villages would join in worship every
Sunday. This type of ritual helped to cement the notion of belonging to
a particular local.

In an everyday sense the traditional market day had a similar function.
Mitchell (1986) suggests that in pre-industrial Britain market day was
combined with worship day. In latter times different areas held different
market days. The market day had a similar function of bringing the
community together. Other rituals that gave a timetable to village life
included the various festivals: dancing around the maypole; religious
walks and parades. These offered the village members the opportunity
to work together to make the event successful. Often they would involve
a relationship between the church and work: the harvest festival could
hold the same purpose as the pagan spring rites where the coming of
summer was celebrated by sacrifice and dance. Such festivals created a
bonding between village members which offered a kind of predictability
within relationships. For example, everyone knew that each other would
be at the harvest festival, to absent oneself would be abnormal. The
rituals and timetables of the 'community' created a group identity which
could be seen as tribalism. Outsiders were viewed with suspicion. Indeed
the Poor Law had legislation to deal with outsiders. In other societies
raids against other tribes are viewed as normal practice. In short there
is security in a group identity. One belongs and is protected against
attack from outside. Rituals are utilized to cement the bonds between
the group members, a process adopted by modern groups, e.g. free-
masons. They advertise that the group exists.

Many groups today bond their members by rituals. Skidmore (1986)
observed rituals of inclusion and exclusion within social groups. These
often manifested by way of ritualistic speech or actions which were
only recognized by those who were members of the group. That group,
however, will have a history, a tradition that is based upon the dynamics
of the wider society. In a sense each group has an institutional context
and, consequently, is humanly produced (Berger and Luckmann, 1984).
Tradition is another safety net that feeds into the security factor for most
human groups. Shared tradition suggests similar roots which in turn
suggest similarities of beliefs and hence predictability. Berger and Luckmann (1984) argue that socialization always takes place in the context of
a specific social structure. We are subjected to the socialization process
from the moment we are born (Schutz, 1962) which suggests that every
aspect of life is socially structured in some way. This social structure is
important to maintain society itself; it contains the code for societal
living. We place honesty as a virtue in western society and yet, as Trevor
(Leland, 1988) suggests, we are afraid of real honesty because it causes
those in power to lose control. We reinforce the honesty that supports

the common good. Most children become the product of the social lie, i.e. not saying what they really think because it is rude.

In this respect we are all children since we have invested confidence in a dishonest structure. We are socialized into believing that the normal world is a safe and secure place rather than being made to face the truth that we are walking along a tightrope from which we can fall at any moment. Everytime a child is murdered we are shocked and outraged because real people do not harm children; everytime a new scandal of sexual perversion is exposed we wonder how people could commit such acts; when the horrors of war are illustrated by the media we are horrified that anyone could allow this to happen. In order to protect the security of our world we explain these acts as those of monsters and madmen. Stereotypes offer security because they permit explanations. Similarly when friendship and love are exposed as false people rarely deny the existence of either but attribute the falseness to the other party (Skidmore, 1986). There is, of course, a danger in maintaining the belief in the security and safety of societal living, it hampers the development of coping strategies.

THE FALSEHOOD OF THE NORMAL SOCIETY

One shared concept between all countries in our Atlas of Existence is that of the 'normal' society. There is a belief that most people live by a code of behaviour that allow us all to co-exist in relative harmony; that there is a natural and just order to the world. To some extent this dictates how we are meant to behave, a concept briefly explored earlier. For instance we are tolerant of certain social errors from children but expect that they will grow out of them; if a person persists in childish behaviours into adult life then we recategorize that person in some way. This allows the rest of us to control him either by providing a reason for the behaviour or by allowing our agents to enforce treatment upon him. Very rarely will we accept that he is an individual who is driving his own path through life. To accept such an explanation would be to threaten the very foundations of society because it would support difference rather than similarity. Difference suggests chaos and unpredictability and works against our social construction of reality. Berger and Luckmann (1984) suggest that we not only understand another's subjective processes but also the world in which he lives and that world becomes ours. Buber (1970) argues to the contrary that we can never understand another's world, merely gain a perception of it. To accept the chaotic existence is to admit that we do not understand the world and, consequently, to lose control.

Consider the intervention of a professional carer; this is based on a theory that seeks to explain the reasons for disease. In order to cope with the world the carer has, by necessity, to devise diagnostic categories which are, in themselves, symbols. A diagnosis says much more than simply what is wrong with a person, it suggests how they came to be in that state and how they should be treated and how long we can expect them to be ill. In a sense the process of diagnosis becomes a structure in its own right and immediately loses sight of the individual. When a person becomes ill they enter a foreign country and, as has been suggested above, being in a foreign country means walking a tightrope high above the ground (Kundera, 1984). The diagnosis becomes the professionals' safety net that seeks to make illness a uniform process. Unfortunately illness is a chaotic process and people react to it in many different ways. However, because the patient is cultured within the falsehood of normality he will interpret his 'unpredictable' response (i.e. he is still feeling pain when the doctors and nurses say he should not) as his condition being worse than suspected; not that the experts may be wrong.

This need to develop categories and classifications is crucial for the development of an Atlas of Existence. The contours are those constellations of agreement that we share with our peers and, consequently, exist on a very public level. Like any atlas many people will have access to it, but some portions will mean more to some than others. The outline of one's own country will signify much more than detailed study of the representation of a foreign country. Similarly few people will have access to many parts of one's personal atlas. Whilst much of the atlas is offered up front (public) there is a very private (backstage) aspect to life (Goffman, 1969). The public aspect will inform us that life is safe and secure; the private may well highlight tightropes over which we are compelled to cross.

Normal life is overstrung with many such tightropes whose existence is denied. The recent media attention given to the abduction and murder of children has led to expressed codes of conducts from the police and other areas of the public sector. Children are told not to go off with strangers; few children would. Many are murdered by people they know ... the very people that the 'normal' society prompts them to trust. At the beginning of this chapter we examined how some of these tightropes have been exposed and subsequently ignored. Marriage is no longer assumed to be for life and alternative relationships are now accepted. However, many members of society still have difficulty in accepting relationships other than the man-wife model. We have witnessed the development of the feminist movement and the rise and fall of the new man, all of which have been used to try and explain the condition of society. To focus on feminism, the worst aspects of gender stereotyping are abhorrent, as is any process that creates structured bias towards any group. However, whilst the academic world is tying itself in knots trying to devise politically correct vocabularies, we are still subjected to gender-specific toys and advertisements. Children are still encouraged, by adults, to enter into gender-specific play. Many girls are cultured into the feminine role by play in that their 'toys' are miniatures of what they can expect in their adult world: plastic babies, plastic cookers and washing machines ... the implication being that they are expected to grow into the 'carers' of society. Fantasy games and aggressive toys are distinctly targetted at the male child.

Similarly there appears to be a significant rise in incidences of sexual harassment in the workplace since the late 1980s. What we appear to lose sight of is that many males have received no instruction in how to relate to the female. However modern the man is sex will always be in the background. Even the modern man is exposed to the stereotyped relationship portrayed through the media: the male hero ends up in bed with the female lead; when central casting creates a beautiful blond for the main role of killer she will tend to use sexual activity to entrap victims. There are no famous films or novels that explore an egalitarian, sex-free relationship between men and women. The media is part of the process of structuring our reality. If the media's message is that both parties are bonded by a mutual interest in sex then the subject will always be on the agenda in male and female encounters.

This text is not seeking to maintain the status quo by justifying acts of sexism or sexual harassment, but it does seek to illustrate that alternative strategies require to be advertised when we attack the existing behaviours. When there was a place for everything and everything in its place we could recognize and feel safe within our community. Now that tightropes are being exposed the world becomes increasingly unsafe for many people. Entering a relationship is one tightrope, being the member of a family is another, gaining employment yet another and we can fall from any or all. Walking a tightrope demands a sense of balance and a confidence in one's own steps. Tightrope walkers tend to know how long the rope is and how far it is from the ground ... the social tightropes are totally unknown. People are different and growing increasingly happy about showing the same; hence, when we step onto the tightrope of a relationship with a member of the opposite sex there are no indications about whether you'll even get onto the rope.

Parents, in order to protect their child's security, have perfected the social lie. The most heinous is surely the retort: you'll know when the time comes. 'When will I know when a girl likes me?'; 'When will I know when I've met the right man?' ... you'll know when the time comes. Knowing is usually based on informed judgement not on hit and miss experiences. Consequently when a girl/boy shows interest instead of spitting at you one assumes the time has come. The social lie reinforces the 'false' normality which fosters a false security in the young. Intravenous drug users and adolescents frequently indulge in risk behaviour because they feel that they know their partners (Skidmore, 1993). Drug

users will share works with other addicts they 'know'; young males
will have unprotected sex with partners they 'know'. With reference to
unprotected sex research suggests that knowing can mean having sex on
the first date without a condom. When people talk of knowing they
really mean projection. In simplistic terms the dynamics are that we
identify a commonality with someone we are attracted to. That commonality may be a sense of humour, but once the connection is made a
person invests all their other qualities into another. In Berger and Luckmann's (1984) terms that person's world becomes a shared world. Hence,
because I am free of sexually transmitted disease so are they and sex is
safe. Witness this description taken from an interview:

Q: Do you have unsafe sex?
R: No . . . never . . .
Q: So you use condoms all the time?
R: I've never used one and never would . . .
Q: But you just said that you never have unsafe sex . . .
R: I don't . . . I only sleep with girls I know.
Q: I see . . . and how long do you know them before . . .
R: Varies . . . sometimes a day or so . . . sometimes it's weeks . . .
Q: A day? How do you know they are safe?
R: You just do . . . don't you? Well you can tell . . .

The delusion of knowing permeates much of societal living. Skidmore
(1986) suggests that many friendships are based on the feeling of knowing rather than real knowledge about the partner. And yet, that feeling
of knowing the world is central to our ability to negotiate a path through
the world. Without a concept of normality there could be no societal life
as we know it. Every encounter would have to be a totally new negotiation and friendships would take many years to establish. In reality
courtships betweeen lovers and friends tend to be relatively short affairs.

THE CONSEQUENCES OF ACCEPTING FALSEHOOD

Berger and Luckmann (1984) offer a succinct and recognizable view of
society:

> Put simply, everyone . . . is what he is supposed to be . . . Everyone
> knows who everybody else is and who he is himself. A knight is a
> knight and a peasant is a peasant, to others as well as to themselves.
> There is, therefore, no problem of identity . . .

For very many people the false security of society is welcome; they
sail through life with few difficulties and experience happiness, which
we all seek. Those who find themselves on the tightropes are in the
minority and will be disadvantaged by how society views them. The fact

that there is a government that we vote for, that there are inequalities in society and that you are reading a book that suggests an ideology of community care indicates that the majority of people accept the falsehood of normality. Normalities, however, are based on majorities and consequently leave little room for the individual. The majority response is factual, i.e. it is an average response within any group; an individual response is actual, i.e. it has been experienced. Problems of identity only occur when one is at odds with the factual. For example, the evidence suggesting that smoking and lung cancer are linked is based on factual evidence. This means that there is an associated relationship between the two variables (smoking and cancer). The data are collected cross-sectionally, which means that the death rates for cancer of the lung and sales of tobacco are collected at the same time in various places (Black *et al.*, 1984). In truth the people who are dead cannot be the same as those buying tobacco. This is why people can offer 'actual' evidence to defend their smoking habit: my Grandma smoked 90 full-strength from the age of 14 and was killed by a bus at 90! Factualities, like norms, are the product of human construction and prone to weaknesses.

The consequences of accepting any falsehood only become problematical if we suffer because of it. The smoker who accepts the 'actualities' and continues to smoke and subsequently develops a chronic lung disease is just as at risk as a member of society who believes that there are lots of safety nets to break his fall. In both cases the person's perception is clouded by his experience of the world and what he wants to believe. The notion that people are merely actors is not new in sociology and social anthropology (Atkinson, 1990). Atkinson (1990) argues that studies that illustrate 'backstage behaviour', or that behaviour viewed as not normal, are more likely to be remembered with a snigger than as major contributions to sociological work. More significant, Atkinson (1990) illustrates that even academics invest in symbolism to project normality and predictability. He refers to titles of studies:

> The use of titles, of course, provides a sign which enters the text into relations with others . . .

Everyday life is full of titles: mother, child, lover and friend. The title places something in context within a wider world. It offers a great deal of information, just as the diagnosis or any form of classification does. Similarly when we accept an actuality we are placing it in reference to ourselves. Just as we can reject the meaning conveyed by a title, because we have read something contrary, so too can we reject the meaning conveyed by someone else's experience . . . because ours is disparate. The point is that we will tend to accept the meaning that makes us more comfortable. If I enjoy smoking I know I will come to no harm because of my experience of my Grandma . . . back to knowing again.

In Chapter 1 the notion of random man was introduced. In essence this is all about chaos since it explores the possibility of a life unfettered by rules, other than to do what one wants to do. This places the individual, rather than the group, in prime position within society. To place one individual above all others is rather anarchic and yet it is what most people do every day of their lives. Social life cannot be read like the contours of a map. Geography is relatively fixed in that we know we can fly to Athens and will see the same landmarks that others have described. We cannot similarly visit someone's life and expect it to be identical to the last time it was visited. Notions of community and society imply this, reality illustrates something quite different. A person is constantly interacting with his society and will change because of that interaction (Banks, 1984). At the same time he is manipulated into portraying a predetermined role by the virtue of his title. The ramifications of that title have been learned through socialization. Because a large part of his display is an 'act' it is possible to witness 'backstage behaviours'. Those backstage behaviours are likely to become problematical to the community if the display is prolonged ... in other words if a person acts himself. In this respect the consequences of the falsehood are to imprison all the actors within the arena.

At the same time the falsehood is very attractive since it offers a sense of belonging and acceptance. The human construction of reality reinforces the group (community) rather than the individual. Governments decree policies that are supposed to be for the common good, and we elect the government and convince ourselves that there is, after all, a democracy. That democracy only exists within a concept of normality and a sense of community. If one introduces individuality then even the safety of government comes under threat. In truth we cannot vote for whosoever we like, our choice is limited to those allowed to stand. In truth, once elected the government decides its own policies with no need for a referendum. In truth we start to recognize Nietzsche's notions of society being the externalization of its greatest men and women.

Naturally most people do not worry about such issues because they are quite comfortable and reassured by the falsehood. Humans are so adept at constructing a meaningful structure around them that stimulating disbelief in community would be very difficult. Self is central to existence and consequently that which self believes becomes paramount. Back to Frankenberg's (1975) suggestion that each person sees himself as the centre of his own social network, one could extend this by suggesting that each individual sees himself as the centre of all existence. Consequently that which offers comfort and security will be adopted. People tend to weave a net of ritual around their lives that offers anchorage for their ideals. To belong and be accepted are essential elements of community life and we find many ways of gathering evidence for belonging.

A person negotiates a route through his social life. It is in his interest to try and conform so that the passage through life is as comfortable as possible. Part of that negotiation involves people gaining more titles that locates them within everyone elses' existence. These titles are far more than role identifications. In many western male groups the use of nicknames indicates that a member belongs to a particular sect. It is, in many ways, an extension of being awarded the colours of a particular tribe.

PUBLIC VERSUS PRIVATE

So far there has been allusion to both a public and private aspect of a person. The concept is not new and has been explored by others (Goffman, 1969; Strauss, 1969; McCall and Simmonds, 1978; Atkinson, 1990). However, the influence of one on the other has been largely ignored. Publicly people develop points of agreement that bond them within a certain network. It has been argued that this sense of agreement offers a feeling of belonging that creates a type of safety net. Conversely it has been suggested that the safety net is based upon falsehoods. Why then, if the latter is true, do millions of people allow their lives to be controlled in various ways? Why do we not just do as we will? In fact, some people do but are punished by the rest of us. The key to understanding why we support the falsity of social life may lie in the private dimension of a person's life. The nature and structure of society has conspired to make man believe that he is here for a purpose, be it to inherit the world or evolve into a new life form. This, of course, is the ultimate comfort and the ultimate form of control. Our 'self' informs us that we are in some way unique and not like any other. We gain reinforcement for these beliefs through evidence that our ideals exist. Those ideals are things like love and friendship. In Chapter 1 it was suggested that people rarely test friendships . . . they know that they exist. Just as the drug users and adolescents know their partners! There are large portions of everyday life which exist in similar ways. The 'knowing' is very much a private thing. What can a person know better than their own secret world? When we mix with others who reinforce the structure of our secret world, even though they are denied access, our sense of belonging is confirmed.

The public and private dimensions, rather than being separate worlds, co-exist in tandem and, at the same time, as a continuum. We may try to keep them apart but they continually impinge on each other. Earlier in this chapter the development of a relationship with a member of the opposite sex was introduced. Research has indicated that couples are capable of maintaining two types of relationship, the public (that with a known partner) and the private (that with a secret lover). Keeping the relationship secret allows both parties to actualize more of their private self within the relationship; in other words to live out one's fantasies. Because the public relationship, such as marriage, is structured through the public life it must conform to the rules we expect that others adhere to, i.e. it must be seen to be normal. Because those in our networks share and agree (or seem to agree) with the structure we cannot break away from the norms without penalization. When relationships break up part of the network changes; divorce is more than losing a partner, one also loses friends. Perhaps this is another aspect of the falsehood of society, that we find it difficult to be totally open with those supposedly close to us. To do so may advertise that we are not who we declared we were and that threatens our location within a network. A relationship with someone outside the network, or someone who is prepared to absent him/herself, cannot threaten the location and, hence, can be subjected to honesty. Research suggests that more people confide intimate secrets to strangers on trains than to close friends (Brain, 1977; Duck, 1983; Miller, 1983; Skidmore, 1986).

To take this further: if society is based on falsehood, then public relationships are similarly based to lesser or greater degrees. Boy meets girl and fantasizes about her but, at the same time, constructs attributes about what she will like in boys (based on his experience). He starts to relate to her and picks up cues on that which she does like and becomes the person they have both constructed. They enter a relationship and marry. In time parts of his private self start to emerge because he tires of 'living his life for someone else'; he is accused of not being the person that she married and they part. In fact he never was the person that she married . . . neither person (bride nor groom) existed in reality. Similarly interviews with secret lovers betray the fact that these relationships fail when attempts are made to 'normalize' them, i.e. make them socially acceptable. In short we are not cultured into the chaotic and try to place the secret relationship within the normal context of 'man-wife'. This theme is very evident in Kundera (1984) where he illustrates how relationships fragment when attempts are made to draw them into a 'normal' structure.

In conclusion, whilst there are positive aspects of belonging to a network it is based on a concept of normality. Normality is group defined and denies the individual; however we are not schooled in being individuals and either subscribe to the network or develop a secret life. Another aspect of the secret life is to fall into fantasy, or to live in one's head, a concept to be explored later. The public and the private often pull a person in different directions, then. The person's culture informs him that humanity is special; his private musings indicate that he is more special, and yet he is incapable of shaping his own life.

In the next chapter we will explore in more detail how the tension between public and private can lead to a person being exiled from his network.

REFERENCES

Ashe, S.E. (1955) Opinion and social pressure. *Scientific American,* **193**(5), 31–55.
Atkinson, P. (1990) *The Ethnographic Imagination,* Routledge, London.
Banks, I. (1984) *The Wasp Factory,* Futura, London.
Berger, P. and Luckmann, T. (1984) *The Social Construction of Reality,* Penguin, Harmondsworth, Middlesex.
Bilton, T. *et al.* (1987) *Introductory Sociology,* Macmillan, London.
Black, N., Boswell, D., Gray, A. *et al.* (1984) *Health and Disease,* Open University Press, Milton Keynes.
Brain, R. (1977) *Friends and Lovers,* Paladin, St Albans.
Buber, M. (1970) *I and Thou,* T. & T. Clark, Edinburgh.
Duck, S. (1983) *Friends for Life: the psychology of close relationships,* Harvester Press, Brighton.
Frankenberg, R. (1975) *Communities in Britain,* Penguin, Harmondsworth, Middlesex.
Goffman, E. (1969) *The Presentation of Self in Everyday Life,* Penguin, Harmondsworth, Middlesex.
Kundera, M. (1984) *The Unbearable Lightness of Being,* Faber and Faber, London.
Leland, D. (1988) *Made in Britain,* Central Independent Television, Birmingham.
Lockwood, D. (1958) *The Blackcoated Worker,* Allen and Unwin, London.
McCall, G.L. and Simmonds, J.L. (1978) *Identities and Interactions: an examination of human associations in everyday life,* Free Press, New York.
Miller, S. (1983) *Men and Friendship,* Gateway Books, London.
Mitchell, J. (1986) Interview, in D. Skidmore: *The Sociology of Friendship,* University of Keele.
Schutz, A. (1962) *The Problem of Social Reality: collected papers,* Martinus Nijhoff, The Hague.
Skidmore, D. (1986) The sociology of friendship: historical, literary and empirical perspectives. University of Keele, PhD Thesis.
Skidmore, D. (1993) Risk behaviour, The Manchester Metropolitan University, unpublished research (on-going).
Strauss, A.L. (1969) *Mirrors and Masks: the search for identity,* The Sociology Press, California.
Young, M. and Wilmot, P. (1957) *Family and Kinship in East London,* Routledge and Kegan Paul, London.
Zinski, J. and Zinski, M. (1973) *The Extra-Marital Arrangement,* Abelard-Schuman, London.

CHAPTER 3

Natives, exiles and refugees

Every country has its natives, those that belong, who share the same language, customs and norms. We have referred to these collections of natives as 'networks' and explored how this very public way of life offers a sense of belonging and of security. Membership, or being a native, of the network is conditional. Immediate entry may be given as part of one's birthright, others may earn the right of admission. A study of male networks has revealed rules of membership (Skidmore, 1986, 1993). Many male networks are bonded by activity (sports or drinking) and there are clear rules of attendance and contribution. Outsiders can join peripheral activities but one is elected to membership once commitment has been proved.

It could be argued that this is a micro-reflection of wider society. One can be born a native but must maintain residence in order to remain a true native. Morris (1967) indicates similar tribalistic rules within human groups. Conforming to the rules and norms of the country is a key element in maintaining membership. Conformity fosters predictability and, as Strauss (1969) suggests, predictability makes relationships stable. Providing a member plays the role he contributes towards the predictability and, hence, the stability of the network. The structure of friendship and association is the very essence of society. They provide functions:

A sense of belonging
Emotional integration and stability
Opportunities to communicate about self
Assistance and physical support
Reassurance of our worth and value
Opportunity to help others
Personality support

(Duck, 1983; Hays, 1984)

Being a native is a relationship of association and association will only survive through shared activity (Skidmore, 1986). Membership through birth, as argued above, has to be reinforced by actions. Birthright only provides a right of access. There are three prominent benchmarks to association:

1. Advertising that one shares the beliefs and attitudes of the group; this draws members into an association pool, or network.

This, over time leads to:

2. Increasing intimacy within the group; access to physical and mental closeness.

Finally:

3. Advertising ... letting members know by rituals of inclusion and others by rituals of exclusion of shared closeness.

(adapted from Duck, 1983)

Hess (1972) stresses this supportive notion of association and sees it as a system of creating and maintaining social reality for its members (the falsehood, Chapter 2). Boissevain (1974) argues that it offers affection and protection. To explore being a native in more depth we can dissect the benchmarks below.

SHARING BELIEFS AND ATTITUDES

The tradition of one's 'culture' has already been explored in Chapter 1. There is a code for life in each network which we learn through social interaction. This creates expectations within the group about how each member should broadly live his or her life. The timetables loosely out-lined in the previous chapters are a part of this. Each member is expected to conform to that timetable; some flexibility will be allowed, but gener-ally members will be expected to reflect agreement to the expectations of them through their actions. For example, in some 'networks' males are expected to 'settle down' by a certain age, 21 for the sake of argument. The network may allow 3 years' variation on either side, but if the member is advertising no intention of 'settling down' by the age of 28 explanations for the non-conformist behaviour will be sought. Often these will originally be prompted by close family members and primarily in jest:

All the nice girls will be snapped up
I'm never going to be a grandmother

The pressure to conform can be even more intense for the female:

You'll end up an old maid ...

Continued failure to conform to the norm will result in the member being reclassified and his/her membership may be called into question.

Those who embrace the rules and are seen to be living a similar life to his/her peers will be afforded the full support of the group. It is these very acts of advertising a shared belief and attitude that is the key to the falsehood of society. We do not need to support a belief or opinion to advertise it. Duck's (1983) analysis of friendship comes unstuck because it was based on reported common attraction: i.e. friends laid claim to sharing similar views to each other. These aspects of relationships are something we can never expose because it would mean members of a network revealing individuality. Consider the Ashe (1955) experiments on conformity . . . the pressure to conform, to be a native, is quite intense.

This is nowhere more apparent than through illness behaviour. If we are declared to be ill then we are expected to act ill. If we refuse to conform to this role then it is not illness or we do not wish to get better. Illness behaviour will be explored in more detail later in the text.

INCREASING INTIMACY

These benchmarks are not clearly segregated parts of a native's career. They are part of a fluid continuum from which a person may move in and out of. Consequently one does not serve a certain amount of time advertising one's conformity before increased intimacy is delivered. This may be implied by the marriage analogy but is in no way intended. For a start most people will belong to more than one network and these may overlap; humans are very resourceful when it comes to insurance. In many ways a person will be unaware that s/he has passed a benchmark until well after the event. When people are asked to explain when a relationship became intimate they have difficulty in recalling precise moments (Skidmore, 1986). However, in order to get the concept over it requires a mechanistic handling.

The native advertises his conformity and over time will find that he is rewarded with much more intimacy within the group. The longer his membership extends the more predictable and secure he becomes to the group. He will be party to developing the shorthand style of speech, giving and receiving nicknames, and enjoy the physical and mental support of the ranks closing round him when he is under threat. Intimacy is a feature of this part of the native's career but will rarely be a group value. It has already been argued that groups marginalize the individual. In association (the network) two or more members will become more intimate at times (the notion of the best friend) and may subsequently slip back to being less intimate (Turner and Turner, 1978). Being a native is an institutional relationship which lacks intimacy per se since it is negotiated within a group context. Intimate relationships are personally defined and often emanate from the private self; consequently they lack institutionalization (Paine, 1969). Often conformity and predictability is confused with knowing. Because people 'act' in the institutional relationships of association we feel that we know them. Nietzsche (1977) suggests that:

... we invent and fabricate the person with whom we associate – and immediately forget we have done so.

However, there are so many rituals to reinforce the 'false' intimacy that 'knowing' one's group overcomes any doubts that we may have. We enjoy belonging. Because we enjoy belonging we are prepared to share some of our secrets with others knowing that we will receive their support.

INCLUSION AND EXCLUSION

These are natural progressions from the above. The act of giving and receiving nicknames affords greater access to mental and physical support, but at the same time it excludes those who do not know who owns which nickname, and it includes the owner of the nickname. Inclusion and exclusion advertise to others the location of the group and the members in it. It is a subtle way of wearing your colours. It was suggested above that it is not really possible to split these into clear categories. There is an element of advertising from the moment a person is born into a culture. His appearance will advertise that he belongs to a certain group, excluding him from others; his language will include him in a wider society, exclude him from many others and locate him regionally. The extremes of exclusivity can be witnessed in racism where qualities of membership include certain members who feel they have more status than others and the attributes of exclusion lead to persecution.

The process of being a native is very much an exchange system. One invests conformity and in return receives membership. Some members may be more important than others, but no single member will be more important than the group. Even though our investment in the group may be based on a set of ideals and myths, we feel that we know the members, that we belong, that we are supported and above all that we are located. This offers a sense of purpose and meaning to the world.

NON-CONFORMITY

Conversely certain persons will refuse to conform. Perhaps because the private dimension is stronger than the pressure to conform a certain class of people ignore the rules. In a sense they do not 'know their place' and defy all attempts that others make to point this out. On a fairly innocuous level it could be the female who refuses to settle down with a family, favouring a career instead. More threatening to society are those females who insist on taking up recognized 'male' occupations (e.g. welding). These females will attract the title of 'tomboy' and in some cases their histories will be rewritten by parents to justify the outcome. At an treme level there is the person who abandons social niceties, has no inhibitions and does as he pleases. Such a person may attract the label of 'deviant'.

Just as one cannot simply lay claim to being a native, similarly one cannot decide to be a deviant. The social web conspires against such declarations by trying to normalize non-conformist behaviours. At this stage we have to remember that the acceptable view of life is one of predictability, of an ordered progression through life. Those who follow a different path must have a similar explanation. What is not allowed for in this steady progression (such as the three benchmarks outlined above) is catastrophic progression: i.e. a sudden change without cues that allow observers to predict the change. We can diagrammatically represent normal social interaction as a two-dimensional continuum. Consider acceptance to rejection:

Acceptance - Rejection

We may even add another dimension here:

Conformity - Non-conformity

and place these on a grid (Figure 3.1):

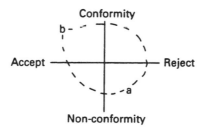

Fig 3.1 Conformity-acceptance grid.

In Figure 3.1, the closer to 'a' a subject is, the more likely it is to be rejected, whereas 'b' has the best chance of being accepted. There will be variations with greater or lesser degrees of acceptance/rejection as one moves around the grid in a steady, progressive way. In reality, however, behaviour can change catastrophically (Woodcock and Davis, 1978). This is represented in Figure 3.2.

The theory illustrated in Figure 3.2 permits the usual natural progression of change (acceptance to rejection, A through D) but suggests more dramatic reactions. For example, one may plunge immediately to rejection (A to D) without gradual progression, as in instant dislike. This is a three-dimensional model rather than a two-dimensional model. The dislike is instant and explains the extreme aspects of racism. Visitors to

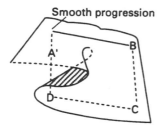

Fig 3.2 Catastrophe graph.

a foreign land may experience this type of rejection. However, it is unlikely that a non-conformist in his own country would experience a similar reaction, providing that he was physically conforming at birth. As has been said above, the first reaction of the immediate network is to attempt to normalize non-conformist behaviour. That is an attempt by fellow natives to offer meaning for the non-conformity. The social web of conspiracy, in this sense, prevents catastrophic reaction.

One should remember that both models offer a bidirectional movement: one can move gradually from rejection to acceptance, or catastrophically. The components of social life are many. Consequently one can be seen as a non-conformist in many ways. In Chapter 1 the dimensions of life were suggested as: social (which we have so far concentrated on), psychological (which has been alluded to), biological and political. Social acceptance is complex because we can be catastrophically rejected in any of these components.

BIOLOGY

This is the aspect over which we have no control; we are born a specific sex, our genes will dictate height, body size and even deformity. Any of these carry with it a social implication since the society one is born into will have had experience of, and developed expectations about, previous biological 'misfits'. Our attractiveness to the opposite and same sex is determined by biology; how we respond to infection and nutrition is also an aspect over which we have little control.

SOCIOLOGY

Our physical appearance will, to some degree, dictate how the society which we are born into reacts towards us. We could be rejected or accepted, the response of those around us will dictate the level of conformity we show. You cannot conform if you are excluded. In this sense the biology and sociology are integrated.

PSYCHOLOGY

This will develop from the private aspects of self and be heavily influenced by the combination of biology and sociology. The strength of the private self will determine how much we struggle against rejection and those strategies we employ to combat same.

POLITICS

In the sociological sense politics is about control. The combination of our biology, sociology and psychology will influence the amount of control we feel we can exert regarding our location. Some will give in and become a victim, others will struggle against the tide.

Again these aspects are not so clear cut but constantly influence the others. For example, it is now generally accepted that when we are under stress (political and psychological dimensions) we can become ill (biological) which will influence our social dimension. Consequently all aspects are interrelated so that a crisis in any one of the dimensions can cause catastrophic changes in the others. Figure 3.3 shows this model developed in a three-dimensional image.

The cut-away of the sociology cube illustrates that each quadrant has a dimension of the other and the biology cube of the larger sociology cube could be similarly represented. This model, then, incorporates Chaos theory (Gleick, 1987) where each major component can be composed of a series of fractals. Gleick (1987) suggests that a fractal is a way of seeing infinity. In the following model the sociology cube would be broken down into four cubes of sociology, biology, psychology and politics; in turn the smaller sociology cube would be similarly broken down and so on. This would also happen for all the other cubes. Each cube contains miniature replicas of itself and all other cubes. In turn, each cube connects with the other cubes; hence, all things are related. A person's life components, then, are suggested to be a collection of interrelated cubes, each one influencing the next. Should anything go wrong with one of the fractals it will in turn cause a ripple effect throughout the whole model. The strength of that ripple will dictate whether catastrophic action occurs.

The influence on the fractal can be three fold: internal (motivated by self), external (motivated by others), natural (motivated by nature/ biology). The combination then is infinite and offers an explanation for the tightrope theory of life.

Phew . . . a little bit heavy. Let us return to the concept of deviance. It has been suggested that one does not merely declare deviance it is just as much negotiated as is normality. Consider the male who has not learned the rules of courtship and attempts to kiss every female he meets.

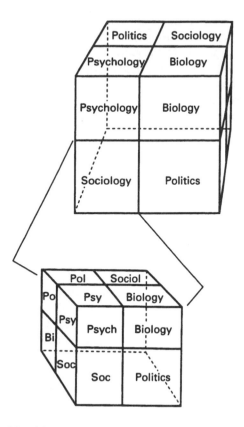

Fig 3.3 Modified health career model. (After Hodges, 1986)

At an early age (e.g. 7 years) it will be explained as him being naturally affectionate. As he grows older he may be labelled precocious until the time arrives when he can no longer be contained within the normality framework. He may then be referred for expert assessment. The expert will classify him according to his theoretical framework. Should the classification suggest that he is sexually deviant, his network will renegotiate his location in relation to that which is normal. In effect he will become an exile from his own country.

Many 'deviants' internally reassess their activities until they are viewed by the deviant as normal. In effect the network is dysfunctive. This can often be reinforced by the immediate family and friends who try to normalize the activities (primary normalization). This is often acceptable if it can be contained within the network. However, more severe cases will be forcibly exiled from the 'community' in hospitals and prisons where they will meet and interact with fellow refugees. This will institute a process of secondary normalization which will reinforce the 'private' belief that such activity is normal. Again, we must remember that societal living is not geared to chaotic or individual behaviours. The 'deviant' may even be subjected to rehabilitative intervention. The literal definition of rehabilitation is 'to restore to previous state' ... but many start out as deviants! In essence what we tend to mean by rehabilitation is to reshape into a socially desirable type.

Rehabilitation programmes can have the effect of turning natives into refugees within their own network. Consequently we can explore two outcomes to non-conformist behaviour: exiles and refugees.

EXILES

Exiles will, by definition, be removed from their network or will voluntarily remove themselves, because of circumstances. Normally an exile is one who is banished by decree. Most societies have mechanisms whereby 'deviants' can be banished. The ancient Athenians called it ostracism since it was the product of a vote. Those members of Athens felt to be gaining too much power or influence (in discord with democracy) could, if a majority voted for it, be banished for up to 10 years (Plutarch, 1961). Our society incorporates a similar system in that we vote for what we consider normal and allow agents to carry out the banishment for us. In our society banishment can have many faces, from forcibly removing a person from society (e.g. to prison) to simply ignoring a person's existence. Just as there can be biological death, there can also be sociological death.

The extreme example of the exile in western society is that of the so-called chronically mentally ill. The behaviour of these people was felt to be so non-conformist that they were exiled to large psychiatric hospitals. The consequence of that banishment was that they had to negotiate membership of a new network and became institutionalized. The literature concerning institutionalization is quite extensive and a simplistic summary would fail to do it justice here. However, it is worth exploring some of the major points in relation to the exile. A person can elect to non-conform as a native when his private self becomes dominant. If he is exiled, however, to the prison or hospital the necessary authorities are empowered to punish him for non-conformity. In an 'ordinary' network the laws that protect the majority also protect the person. Witness the rise of vigilante groups in the UK during the early 1990s. These groups were warned that they would be prosecuted if caught. To circumvent the legal agents is seen to be just as deviant as breaking the law, even though the vigilante may mirror the punishment that the legal processes would carry out.

Some networks are seen to be deviant by the wider society. The world of the secret agent or the criminal for instance. Many criminals, however, grew up in a network where such activities were viewed as normal

(Richardson, 1991). Indeed, whilst on the run from prison Richardson (1980) was prompted to write to *The Guardian* explaining that his criminal activities were the normal result of his subculture and that referral to outside agencies such as the police and courts would have been viewed as deviant. This presents us with a major problem because it presents two, well-entrenched, views of normality which are in opposition. The culture which produced the Krays and the Richardsons also produced equivalent codes to that of the wider society. In this sense going to prison would be seen as an occupational hazard for many criminals. Being an exile in this context is more like being an emigre (i.e. exiled because of circumstances but with a fixed belief that one is right and, once circumstances change, one will return to the same network). The emigre endures because he knows the period of exile will end. Other exiles become refugees (Burgess and Maclean for example) and we will explore this further in a moment.

It has been suggested above that one cannot merely become a deviant, there is a process of legitimizing, as illustrated in Figure 3.4.

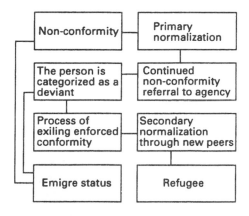

Fig 3.4 Processing the deviant.

Like all other titles the deviant label implies a role set, a certain kind of behaviour about which we can make predictions. In essence the deviant becomes stigmatized. Embodied in the stigmatizing process is a loss of rights since we allow other agencies to inflict a code of conduct onto him. In many ways he has become less than human. Because the process is legitimized we lose sight of the inhumanity we allow our agents to inflict on this group of people. This aspect will be further explored in the chapter concerning government and policy.

Holding institutions such as prisons and hospitals are strictly speaking parts of the 'community', although most authors tend to separate them. You can be exiled from your normal lifestyle into a holding institution and, should you return, you will carry the stigma of the holding institution with you. Let us consider the plight of those people decanted from the psychiatric institutions, after years of exile there, to the 'community'. The years of exile have caused these people to develop predictability from the regulations of the respective institution. Suddenly it is all pulled away. They were offered little choice in the process because government policy was against choice. We can all pontificate that it is fairer because they stand a better chance of being integrated into society. In fact we have caused them to change status from exile to refugee.

REFUGEES

A refugee is one who, owing to religious persecution or political troubles, seeks refuge in a foreign land. The person decanted into the community fits into this role perfectly. A change in belief systems within the professions has led to his persecution and political intervention has reinforced that. This person cannot be rehabilitated because his previous networks, and with them his previous existence, have ceased to exist. To reiterate the point made in Chapter 1 he is in a foreign country, walking a tightrope high above the ground without the safety net afforded to the natives, who have families, colleagues and friends (Kundera, 1984). In addition he is expected to know the rules without instruction. In short he is given a freedom which is more confining than the imprisonment of the institution. That confined freedom is carried in their deportment and etched in their faces. The only security afforded them is to construct a mini-institution within the 'community', in the group home, hostel or public lavatory where most of their day-time shelter is gained. This is hardly integration. Indeed, we have enforced these people into a state of anomie (normlessness). When people enter such a state they are susceptible to suggestion (either external or internal). Society is responsible for this in that we previously removed these people from one network and inflicted them into a rigid regimen. At least they can gain some sense of predictability from this, which society has previously stressed the importance of. However, after 20 years or so it is all suddenly removed. With no social construction the anomie rapidly develops into crisis and any suggestion can be followed (Davis, 1963; Caplan, 1964; Marris, 1974). That suggestion may emanate from the private world and instruct you to jump in front of a train, jump into a lion's den or kill someone.

When such activities become fairly numerous non-conformity is suspected again and we lobby for even more powers for the agents. Several remedies have been suggested for this group of people: special powers for community nurses so that the person can be effectively placed under house arrest; powers to enforce treatment in the community and now powers to have people admitted to hospital. The process of 'caring' may have come full circle but at what price to the individual? Their rights have been totally eroded. Because these people have not been successfully integrated they could all now be forced back into hospital. This process will be further explored in Chapter 5 which discusses government.

The next chapter will explore the concept of the tourist: those persons who visit other countries and momentarily touch the lives of the natives. We can recognize these by their titles: social worker, general practitioner, community nurse and so on.

REFERENCES

Ashe, S.E. (1955) Opinion and social pressure. *Scientific American*, **193**(5), 31–55.

Boissevain, J. (1974) *Friends of Friends: networks, manipulations and coalitions*, Blackwell, Oxford.

Caplan, G. (1964) *Principles of Preventative Psychiatry*, Tavistock, London.

Davis, F. (1963) *Passage Through Crisis*, Bobbs Merril, Indianapolis.

Duck, S., (1983) *Friends for Life*, Harvester, Brighton.

Gleick, J. (1987) *Chaos*, Sphere, London.

Hays, R.B. (1984) The development and maintenance of friendship. *Journal of Social and Personal Relationships*, **1**(1), 75–98.

Hess, B. (1972) Friendship, in *Ageing and Society, vol. 3: a sociology of age stratification*, (eds M.W. Riley, M. Johnson and A. Fowler), Russell Sage, New York.

Hodges, B.E. (1986) *The Health Career Model*, The Manchester Metropolitan University.

Kundera, M. (1984) *The Unbearable Lightness of Being*, Faber and Faber, London.

Marris, B. (1974) *Loss and Change*, Routledge and Kegan Paul, London.

Morris, D. (1967) *The Naked Ape*, Cape, London.

Nietzsche, F. (1977) *A Nietzsche Reader*, Penguin, Harmondsworth, Middlesex.

Paine, R. (1969) In search of friendship. *Man*, **4**(4), 505–24.

Plutarch (1961) *Plutarch's Lives*, Dent, London.

Richardson, C. (1980) *The Guardian*, 29 May.

Richardson, C. (1991) *My Manor*, Sidgwick and Jackson, London.

Skidmore, D. (1986) The sociology of friendship. University of Keele, PhD Thesis.

Skidmore, D. (1993) Risk behaviour, The Manchester Metropolitan University, unpublished research (on-going).

Strauss, A.L. (1969) *Mirrors and Masks*, The Sociology Press, California.

Turner, V. and Turner, E. (1978) *Image and Pilgrimage in Christian Culture*, Blackwell, Oxford.

Woodcock, A. and Davis, M. (1978) *Catastrophe Theory*, Penguin, Harmondsworth, Middlesex.

CHAPTER 4

Tourists, daytrippers and visitors

Should you live in a beauty spot or a place made famous by some television programme there will be certain times of the year you will find trying – the tourist season. Hoards of strangers flocking into your home ground, interfering with your everyday life, clogging the roads and asking lots of questions:

Is this the right road to . . .?
Where do I find . . .?
Is it true that . . .?

Even worse they feel that they have a right to be there because they are paying; more right than the locals and after all it is only for a short time. Well if it was not for tourists where would the economy be?

These troublesome hoards descend onto the landscape vaguely aware of the landmarks, directed by maps (often out of date), with preconceived ideas fostered by listening to friends and travel programmes and with dialects often difficult to understand. Their motive for intruding on your world is self-interest; to gain new experiences and see new sights, or because they enjoyed it/did not see everything last time they were here. The exercise has been designed to fit in with their lives not the natives. Naturally the natives expect them and make some preparations, such as avoiding certain locations at certain times. Whatever preparation is made it cannot be disputed that the lives of the natives are restricted by the tourists. They rush to your favourite places and take snapshots so that they can keep a memory of places. The main thing about snapshots is that they are two dimensional and give a very flat picture of the original. A photograph can never reveal the history underlying a building or place.

The tourist is guided through his Cook's Tour of your world by various guides: road maps and walkways for example. These are designed to illustrate the main features of a particular place and often neglect the finer detail. The tourist's time is valuable, however, so the finer detail is less than important . . . well maybe next year. If they are unsure about the direction the map is taking them they may ask a local, but each has difficulty understanding the dialect of the other. This can lead to misunderstanding and the tourist going off in completely the wrong direction with the local left scratching his head. Then, of course, there is the worst of all tourists . . . the slightly informed know-all who professes to know all about your homeland.

> Of course these barrows were built by the saxons so that they could light beacons on them to warn of attacks from the vikings . . . oh, yes and that Stonehenge was built by Welsh Druids to celebrate Joseph of Arimethea's visit to Wells cathedral . . .

You could try correcting him and pointing out that barrows were ancient burial mounds and that . . . but he'll just wave you into silence, shrug to his friends and carry on believing his own version of history. Tourists are problematical because they pay to visit your homeland and feel that they are helping you by their visits. Still, they do spend a lot of money.

Daytrippers can be worse. Not in terms of feeling they have a right to come and go as they please, like the tourist, but because they want to fit so much in to one day. They fit into two categories: coach tours and small parties. The coach tour may be a mystery tour or a school trip: one lot having no idea where they are and the others not sure why they are there. The small parties (from one to six) at least are interested. However, all of the daytrippers have to rush around to see everything. In the end places become a blur and they are unsure what they have and haven't seen. When their photographs are developed their memories are such a blur they may even wrongly title the snaps. The daytripper may be slightly more informed about the features of your homeland and could be motivated by a real interest. Unfortunately if they have come to visit the local ruins out of interest then they will not spend much money. The coach tours usually come on special rates.

Expected visitors arrive with a different motive. They are coming to see you specifically rather than your homeland. They believe that they want to see you and that you want to see them. Their visit is often pre-arranged and you will be aware of the time and date of their arrival and, if you are lucky, their intended departure. Because you know they are coming to visit you, you have to make a special effort to tidy your surroundings and dress reasonably smartly . . . after all you do not wish to reveal your private self to a visitor, and anyway, it is expected that one makes an effort. They arrive, you make polite conversation, entertain for an hour or so; they ask polite questions that advertise their interest in you but nothing too threatening. Eventually they leave and you are left wondering why they came in the first place.

Unexpected visitors are far more threatening; they arrive unannounced so that you have had no time to prepare the surroundings. Part of your private world may be exposed. They feel no need to apologise because they believe that you are glad to see them ... and because they have this belief they take liberties with your time and sensitivities. It is this type of visitor that makes you decide to hide under the table when you next see them walking down your path.

Tourists, daytrippers and visitors, what have they to do with the theme of this text? Like other titles they present images and most readers will have their own image of each. You may even have insider views and at this moment be ranting that you are not that type of tourist, daytripper or visitor. Unfortunately we all feel that we are not ... and yet someone is for the image to be conjured. Like all groups this class of people suffer from a stereotyped image that picks out the main features of several, say tourists, and creates a composite picture in an attempt to describe all tourists. It does not help that the tourist is always intruding on someone's homeland; no amount of politeness will erode the stereotyped image from the native's mind.

Practitioners are similar to tourists, daytrippers and visitors in that they intrude on a person's geography of being from time to time. We can loosely compare hospital staff to the tourist, community staff to the day trippers and community therapists/voluntary carers to the visitors. Each of these practitioners will carry something of a stereotyped image into the client's world.

People carry their world with them ... they cannot leave it at home when they venture out into a new arena. It is their sense of security and belonging. The exile and refugee may eventually have his world deconstructed over a long period, but for most of us our worlds will withstand limited intrusion. The world of medical and social care is fairly well defined and most natives have cognizance of it. We can break this world into three basic zones:

1. The Lay Lands.
2. Medical Margin.
3. Medical Metropolis.

(modified from Skidmore, 1979)

The Lay Lands

The Lay Lands are normally entrenched within our homelands. We recognize landmarks where we can gain useful information about medical/welfare matters. These landmarks usually manifest as knowledgeable natives: friends, relatives and neighbours. In addition the Lay Lands are constantly informed by the media. If one considers this in terms of having a headache we will either have preparations within the home or we will know how to acquire some. The knowledge of the management of a headache will have been developed over many years. Parents may have modelled headache management, we witness advertisements on the television, see packages in the chemist. In short for what might be termed everyday disorders we will have familiarity with the terrain that allows us to get by. Indeed, it appears that people tend to classify illnesses into two types: that which can be self managed and that which requires assistance (Richman and Skidmore, 1980). Self management depends on the knowledge available. Consider that a person awakes to discover he has a headache. For the first hour or so he may ignore it and involve himself in assessing the likely cause: is it due to too much drink? did I bang my head last night? is the pollen count high? If it persists he will perhaps go to his private supply of medicines (the medicine cabinet in the bathroom or a special drawer) and take the amount of his preferred analgesic that he prescribes. His experience informs him that this usually does the trick. If, however, the headache persists and is still present after several doses he may seek advice from one of his informed natives. The informed native, other than having some knowledge, will also have a range of preparations available. These are usually compiled from uncompleted drug regimens that the person has been prescribed. The range of advice is potentially varied, but at this stage all that is required is consensus with his private view that there is nothing really wrong.

Normally such consensus is arrived at, but from time to time the media alerts the informed natives that all is not right with the world. There have been, for example, several cases of meningitis in the homelands and one has to be careful. The informed native's advice is that one's doctor should be consulted just to be on the safe side. All this time the headache has suggested to the person that he might be ill. Consulting the general practitioner (GP) does not change this. If the advice from the informed native is followed the person will still be on safe ground and still think that he might be ill.

The Medical Margin

The Medical Margin usually overlaps with many peoples' atlas of existence. The central character is the GP about who much is assumed. Skidmore (1979) suggests that most people feel that they know (that word again) their GP. Given that the average person visits their GP at least once every 2 years this is hardly surprising. A person of 30 may have seen him 15 times and will feel that he can make predictions about the encounter:

> He'll probably give me a prescription, tell me to have a few days off work and I'll be alright in a few days.

This expectation will be based partially on the experience of self, partially on the shared knowledge from the Lay Lands and partially on the portrayal of GPs by the media. In short the GP will carry a stereotyped image with him to every encounter. It is not usually GPs who appear on the television news and documentaries warning of deadly diseases. GPs are friendly fellows in the image of Finlay and offer friendly advice. Furthermore a person chooses to consult because he might be ill. The consulting room (or health centre) is usually within the known country and the likelihood is that other known natives will be waiting there. Hence it is a choice encounter, one does not travel too far, one might be ill and one will have definite expectations of what to expect. Nine times out of ten those expectations will be realized. What, then, if the GP refers to a specialist.

The Medical Metropolis

The Medical Metropolis is the capital of matters medical. A referral informs a person of several things:

- one is ill;
- one has no choice of referral;
- one will have to travel (normally);
- it is unknown;
- one has no idea of what to expect;
- hospitals deal with very serious diseases.

In the UK only about a third of the population ever visit a hospital for one inpatient stay. This suggests that the arena is not as well known to the Lay Lands and the Medical Margin. The Lay Lands will be required to draw knowledge from the media and myth. Hospitals are always the centre of drama on the television, life-saving actions are going on all the time and sometimes the actions do not work. Following the referral the person, now well into a patient career, will start seeking reassurance from those in the Lay Lands. Some hospitals will already have a mystique about them, an image which informs. Some hospitals are, for example, noted for their work with cancer. The best example of sensitive planning in the UK is how all the old workhouses were transformed into hospitals for the elderly; the very group who remembered what the workhouse stood for. It was seen to be worse to be sent to the workhouse than it was to be admitted to an asylum. Thus, some hospitals present an image. The apprentice patient seeks reassurance from the informed natives and is offered heart-warming snippets such as:

> Oh, you're seeing Dr Smith . . . that's him who saw my brother just before he died.

Even worse is the motor mechanic reaction: that is when you inform a person which doctor you are seeing and they simply purse their lips, draw breath over their teeth and shake their head. Then there are the horror stories about the hospital:

Isn't that the place where they amputated that chap's good leg and he died because they left the bad one on?

My mother went to have her wisdom tooth taken out there and they dislocated the whole of her lower jaw.

This information will be taken to the encounter by the person. In time a card arrives through the post instructing the person to go directly to the outpatient department several miles away, take the day off work, do not pass go and do not rearrange the appointment. In the UK every outpatient attends expecting to wait at least 2 hours. It is an unknown area, even if it does overlap with the homeland. Being sent there confirms that one is ill and one starts to feel and act ill by the time they arrive. They pass signs that offer cues of severity: mortuary, X-ray and theatres, and then move into a waiting area where other very sick strangers are waiting to be seen. Once seated a person dare not move in case one's name is called and one fails to hear it. Eventually the big moment arrives, one is led into the consulting room which offers more clues about what might happen. The specialist says something but one is so concerned about what might be said one fails to hear what is said. Finally the penny drops . . . one is to be admitted for tests.

If life were a movie it is at this moment when the dramatic music would start. Tests . . . that means cancer does it not? They always say tests when they mean cancer. Of course they also say tests when they suspect anaemia or diabetis but these are not the outcomes that have become entrenched in the Lay Lands data banks. A person will now use all his resources to gauge the severity of his condition. If he is to be admitted immediately then it is very serious . . . if he is to be put on a waiting list, or advised to go private it is relative minor/easy. Tests usually suggest urgency in the Lay Lands, hence that sick-demeanor that the person adopted en route to the hospital is carried back to the home. There is confirmation of illness, no expectations about outcome . . . a loss of power. The person is about to be deluged by tourists; i.e. hospital staff.

THE PRACTITIONER TOURIST

At the beginning of this chapter an image of the tourist was outlined that suggested he visited foreign places out of self-interest, with a clear idea of the landmarks he wanted to see and guided by basic maps. He will take snapshots of these places for future reference. In a similar vein the practitioner tourist, be it hospital doctor, nurse or occupational therapist enters into the professional equivalent. She (the practitioner) is there by virtue of self-interest, that is what prompted the education and training. Because a patient is referred for a specific condition the practitioner has a clear idea of what she expects to see and how to deal with it and will have been directed by the relevant map (theory subscribed to, e.g. the medical model). The assessment (photographs) will be conducted on this premise so that a two-dimensional picture of a person will emerge. The condition becomes paramount rather than how a person might react to a condition.

Unkind, unkind . . . an obligatory swing at the medical model some readers scream. Unfortunately the same is true of the so-called person-centred approaches. Again they are based on group responses (composites and stereotypes) rather than individuals. This has been necessary because if one accepts the individual then, in a population of 57 million, there are 57 million definitions of pain or depression or disaffection. To complicate matters we can never experience another's world (Buber, 1970), which suggests that empathy is not really possible. In addition the therapist will have her special interests and skills and may see what she wishes to see (albeit unconsciously). Unfortunately it is a fact of life that we are all cultured into stereotyping. Professionals are just as guilty as lay people. In practice the consequences of this can be diluted by supervision; i.e. having another professional review your work and question your motives (more of which later).

To return to generally denigrating the actions of practitioners: one should remember the words of C.S. Lewis (1971) '. . . human all too human'. We, in our guise as laiety, expect practitioners to be better than human. We lose sight of the fact that they originated from the same insecurity, were subjected to the same tightropes as the rest of us. Like us they rely on the security of their atlas of existence. Remember this? (Figure 4.1).

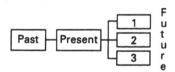

Fig 4.1 The conservative impulse.

Professionals need predictability as well. When they encounter a problem in the present they refer to their education and training to pick up cues about how to deal with the situation. In addition they look around in the present (carry out an assessment) to reinforce their view. Like the rest of us they stereotype and '. . . define first and then see . . .' (Lippman, 1922). That is they see the landmarks that they anticipated. A further complication is their use of language. They introduce a different dialect to the person's world. Skidmore (1981) uses this example when describing the doctor-patient encounter:

Well Mr Smith, the reason you can't walk very far is that you have stricture in the left paraventral guttering.

Cameron (1980) makes similar use of the jargon to make a point and Illich (1976) suggests that this makes medical staff almost priest like. However, if we return to the themes explored in earlier chapters this type of behaviour is quite normal in any group. One grows accustomed to a certain style of speech . . . it offers a sense of belonging. Eventually it becomes so commonplace to the user that they are unaware that misunderstanding can arise. At the same time there is the notion that to speak in 'abstruse' ways gives the impression of being knowledgeable.

Thus far we can witness many of the stereotyped attributes of the tourist being present in the practitioner. Even though the client/patient comes to them he is still bringing his world with him and the practitioner is the intruder. Rituals did exist to make the patient feel like the visitor: the standard bath on admission, changing into bedclothes and being labelled with a condition rather than a name. In recent years there has been a dramatic change to free up the hospitals: wearing one's own clothes, open visiting and being allowed to send out for food. This has had the effect of reinforcing the 'inmates' world. However, what cannot be escaped from is the fact that practitioners are seen as experts. A person is 'cultured' into being passive when ill. Confirmation of illness pushes a person into that zone where they can no longer self-manage, but need help.

Like all things, it is not as simple as the above explanation – a person gets positive aspects from being ill. Parsons (1956) described the ideal type of sick role. The ideal type means that it does not refer to a person specifically, but offers a picture of likely responses. That ideal type suggests two rights and two obligations:

- the right to be absolved from any, or all, obligations;
- the right to receive care and attention.

The sick person is obliged to:

- seek treatment as soon as possible;
- comply with treatment.

Honouring the obligations advertise that one wants to get well. From an early age, however, we learn that there are positive aspects to 'recognized' illness. We are allowed to say no without meaning no:

You can't do the garden with your back

or

You can't go to school like that –

The important point is that the suggestion of illness must come from

someone other than the sufferer. Many people take Parsons (1956) liter-
ally and yet it is quite clear that he intended his view of the sick role to
be a negotiated process (Figure 4.2). Just as in deviance one cannot
merely declare illness, it is a three-way process: the person has to report
the illness, a legitimizing agent (doctor) has to acknowledge the illness
and significant others (natives) have to allow him to be ill.

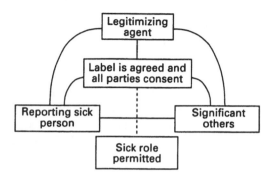

Fig 4.2 The sick role process.

The patient, then, arrives at the hospital and is subjected to numerous
sightseeing experiences: doctors, nurses, students and so on. He is still
very much in his own country and has visitors to reinforce his borders.
The tourists keep invading his country attempting to gain information
about the main features and, like tourists, assume that the patient is
thankful because he is being helped. The authority invested in the tourists
in this arena can permit them to license daytrippers and visitors into a
patient's home upon discharge.

DAYTRIPPERS AND VISITORS

The problem for most community practitioners is that they were cultured
in a tourist environment (the institution) and believed that the world
was theirs. Within the hospital everything is geared to the group: same
mealtimes, medication times and so on. Because the timetable is the
institutions the implication is that it is a separate world. It has already
been suggested that many researchers and writers keep them apart. For
patients the tourists in their world cause restrictions ... they are not yet
exiles or refugees. They have to change their lifestyles until the season
ends. Their experiences of the tourists will colour their images for future
encounters. The community practitioner (for the sake of simplicity,
female), then, is licensed to visit the 'client' at home. She takes with her
an institutional past and the image of representing the tourist. Like the
daytripper she may have several 'clients' to see and so her time is

valuable. Like the daytripper her view of the client will be clouded by her motive; it could be the equivalent of a school trip or genuine interest in the condition.

It is important to understand that both parties will bring their own world to the encounter; both will have clear expectations and images of what is to happen. These images can dictate the direction of the encounter. Let us suppose that the practitioner has arrived to carry out the first discharge visit, postoperation. The operation carried out was fairly routine and she anticipates no problems so has allocated a few minutes for the visit. The client has been home 2 days, slipped in the bath and felt something 'give' during the fall . . . as though the wound had ripped open. The practitioner is expecting nothing sensational, the client is reluctant to reveal his accident (he/she might have been doing something he/she should not have). During the encounter the client senses that the practitioner is in a hurry and so reports nothing. The practitioner writes up the 'snapshot' in a way that suggests that everything is alright. The client gains the impression that the daytripper is not really interested in him, as a person and so merely goes through the mechanisms during future encounters.

Then there is the daytripper who has a personal interest. The history may be along these lines:

> Mrs Jones had a very interesting career prior to having children. She made a decision to give up her career while the children were young and return to work once they started school.

Mrs Jones in fact became an exile because of circumstances. Her own timetables were superseded by those of her children and that of her husband. Her original timetable had involved her career.

> When the children started school Mrs Jones discovered that, due to the recession, she was no longer able to find work. Her identity as the major person in her children's lives is now being threatened by the prominence of teachers: Miss says I can do this . . .

Another part of Mrs Jones identity is being threatened, her career as a mother appears to be moving in the same direction as her career.

> Like others who lose their security Mrs Jones starts entering a period of normlessness. This may manifest as mild depression or irritation. Her husband notices the change in behaviour and suggests that she go and see the doctor.

There is already an implication that she must be ill. Her husband has been used to coming home to a reasonably contented wife for the last 7 years. Suddenly, it seems to him, she has changed and there must be an explanation for it. He suggests that they go out for the evening but she does not feel like it.

> Mrs Jones goes to see the GP and informs him that she is feeling agitated. He prescribes a mild tranquillizer, but has little time to listen in depth (he is a visitor who manages to take a snapshot). The prescription is recorded in the notes and Mrs Jones is informed to return in 2 weeks if she feels no better. She returns, because nothing has changed, and reports that she feels less agitated but now feels depressed. The GP prescribes a mild antidepressant and asks her to return in 2 weeks if she feels no better. Mrs Jones starts feeling really unhappy with her life and now finds that she cannot sleep . . . she returns to her GP . . .

Earlier in this chapter it was suggested that people feel that they know their GPs, similarly they feel that he knows them (Skidmore, 1979). In fact, GPs report that they rarely know patients but do know the notes; once they see the notes they can put a face to them. In the above case Mrs Jones has already gained a psychiatric history. The GP has seen her on three occasions and she has not really responded to treatment, he has only one course of action left: to refer her to a specialist. The consequences are that it confirms to Mrs Jones and her family that she is ill. How the GP actually reports the case will very much depend on how the tourists view her. Rosenhan (1973) reported how specialists responded more to labels than to client's own reports.

In this chapter the interaction between would-be carers and clients have been explored in the context of tourists, daytrippers and visitors. An attempt has been made to illustrate the background that each brings to the encounter. In the next chapter the influence of government, funding and policy will be explored.

REFERENCES

Buber, M. (1970) *I and Thou*, T. and T. Clark, Edinburgh.
Cameron, J. (1980) The pump, unpublished play, broadcast: Yorkshire Television, 6 February 1980.
Illich, I. (1976) *Limits to Medicine*, Penguin, Harmondsworth, Middlesex.
Lewis, C.S. (1971) *Undeceptions*, Bles, London.
Lippman, W. (1922) *Public Opinion*, Macmillan, London.
Parsons, T. (1956) *Social Systems*, Free Press, New York.
Richman, J. and Skidmore, D. (1980) Children's perceptions of health and illness, The Manchester Metropolitan University, unpublished research report.
Rosenhan, D.L. (1973) On being sane in insane places. *Science*, **179**, 250–8.
Skidmore, D. (1979) Anxiety in medical arenas, Cranfield Institute of Technology, MSc Dissertation.
Skidmore, D. (1981) *The Hidden Machine*, Verus, Bournemouth.

CHAPTER 5

Politics, policies and people

Previous chapters have emphasized that in most societies the populace have agents who administer their society on behalf of the majority. These agents constitute a form of government, that is directing the affairs of state. The government in western society is an institution and like any other institution functions for its own purpose rather than having regard for the individual. It is a mechanistic organization – one talks of the wheels of government – rather than humanistic. In societies where people elect government members there is a general notion that the populace have some control over government by the power of the vote. It is the ethic of consensus: if a person feels that they have taken part in the decision-making process then they are more committed to that decision (Gellerman, 1974). To reinforce this ethos people are encouraged to support various parties (Tory, Labour, Republican, Democrat) which supports the consensus notion. If they do not agree with the party in power they are in opposition and in agreement with the opposing party. Democracy as we experience it is another falsehood. Democracy is government by the people; in modern times the codicil '... or their elected agents' has been added. In the strict sense every policy would be decided by referendum. Obviously this would be time consuming and impractical for the smooth working of society. The only effective way to administer a society, then, is through representatives.

Similarly administering large groups (institutions) can only be practical if it serves the majority and it is the majority that have the power of electing. There is then bias in-built into this structure since it places value on the majority over the minority. Similarly a blurring occurs with regard to who the majority are. In the UK government is elected for 5-year periods. Leading up to the election period the people become important and are actively wooed through the media and at the hustings. However, once the election day is passed and the government in seat the need to woo disappears. There are others, however, who have positions of great influence; the leaders of industry, for example, who control much of the economy of the country. If such people are opposed to government issues they could cause a great deal of difficulty for the government. Hence, an influential factor as powerful as the vote emerges, that of economy.

Marx (1955) argued that those who owned the means of production controlled the society and went on to argue that this created a class division in society. His notion of class was far too simplistic in that it is far more complex than simple divisions based on Operators (the controllers) and Things (those being controlled). Weber (1949) was closer to the mark when he introduced the concept of status position. However, there is another crucial factor that creates divisions in society, that of saleability. In any institution economic survival becomes paramount and leads to the organization being led by the need to balance the books. In terms of a large society that taxes earnings this places greater worth on the earners and potential earners. Those who do not earn place a burden on society. That notion of contributors being of more value to society permeates many cultures: the natives of the frozen north used to cast the elderly adrift on ice floes when they lost their faculties; the natives of the new world would will themselves to die when they were no longer useful to the tribe. In western society that contribution is rated on earning power and wealth. The more you earn and save the more you contribute in taxes which oils the wheels of government. Those who no longer earn (the unemployed and the elderly) make claims on those contributions in the shape of welfare benefits.

The NHS was developed for an expanding workforce. The concentration of health care was for workers and prospective workers (the newborn and children). The notion of care from cradle to the grave has never been realized in an egalitarian sense. Since it has been government led, the emphasis on care delivery has been towards those seen to be of greatest value and that has meant acute care. However, because of increasingly better social conditions people are living longer, the longer one lives the more prone to chronic conditions which make greater demands on the NHS. Similarly when people live longer they cost more in welfare benefits (pensions). Economically, by the year 2000, the welfare state in the UK will become inviable in its current state. Those making demands on the state will outweigh those contributing to it (Black *et al.*, 1984). This situation has been compounded by the image of wealth contributing to worth; that is that people feel the more they are paid the more worth they have in society.

Practitioners in the NHS have constantly lobbied for more pay and received the support of the public because they do provide worthwhile roles and valued services. This presents problems for those who control the finances since the amount of money received is finite. Only a finite number of people contribute to the tax pool, and that number is falling because of the recession, but an increasing amount of people are claiming benefits. A portion of those taxes collected are allocated for health and welfare, but these have to pay salaries, services and benefits. If salaries increase the paymasters have limited choices: reduce services, reduce the number of staff, reduce benefits or increase taxes, all of which could threaten the government's electibility. There are, however, other options: we could introduce a cheaper type staff that carries out the same function as existing staff; similarly one could encourage private pensions and redirect the emphasis of care away from caring for the chronically ill to acute care. Caring for the chronic cases could always be placed in the hands of relatives.

The art of fooling most of the people most of the time lies in planning and staged implementation. Consider you have a finite budget which you know is going to be inadequate in 20 years time. To avoid castigation you have to be seen to administer the same service and at the same time delegate the blame, pass the buck. First of all we introduce a scheme of general management. Reorganize the NHS districts into general management units and bring in managers used to managing industry. These general managers will be on fixed term contracts renewable in relation to achievement. The next move is to erode the largest group who make demands on salaries – the nurses. Project 2000 is a great way into this because it offers student nurses real student status. This has a dual spin off:

1. It makes them supernumerary so that the service will develop a system of coping without the extra hands.
2. It affords the opportunity to devolve the training budget to a more local level and thereby give each region the responsibility for its own training for the future. In fact this is such a good idea we will do it for all professions allied to medicine. Transfer the health training aspects from the Department of Education (at 1989 levels) to regions and give them the responsibility. This makes savings on the education budget and the tendering exercises involved will cause the closedown of some smaller colleges, more savings. Added to this is the fact that those regions who did not train certain staff in 1989 get no funds to continue training.

To reinforce these changes we publish our plans for the future in *Working for Patients* (HMSO, 1989), which will offer each unit manager (be that region or trust) to employ the type and number of staff they feel to be appropriate for delivery of care. In the background we fund a body called the National Health Service Training Authority who will produce packages to train staff, on the job, at a basic level and at the same time introduce a concept of Health Care Assistants who will be there only to assist nurses, occupational therapists and other practitioners (honest).

Next we address the issue of Care in the Community. It is everyone's right to receive this kind of care and a veritable scandal that the mentally ill and persons with learning disabilities have been incarcerated for many years. Also if GPs and dentists received their own budgets based on their patient lists they could buy the services their patients need more effectively and efficiently. In this way we can transfer care from government base to localities. To take it further those community nurses – there are a lot of them, aren't there? If we had one generic nurse who supervised health care assistants in specialist areas . . . but softly, softly catchee monkey. To concentrate on the transfer of care, it is relatively easy, because the population invests a sense of worth in certain groups. Young, workers, old, disabled, chronically ill, psychiatric and learning disabilities as a pecking order. When GPs have their own budgets the problems are transfered because GPs will be penalized for overspending . . . hence they will have to select membership of their lists very carefully. The rhetoric surrounding the last two groups in the pecking order will reinforce the plan to reduce the services for them. We transfer these into the community with no equivalent transfer of funds and we can then deconstruct the institutional provision (large savings on buildings and staff). The perceived motive for the transfer is altruistic . . . after all these people should not be stigmatized by different treatment. Hence the special schools and units within schools for those with learning disabilities should be scrapped . . . these children should go through the normal school system in a process of normalization.

The implementation of the deconstruction process for these two groups will be a good pilot for the larger group targetted – the elderly. We can increase the retirement age gradually, that way more people will die in work and never claim a pension. Secondly we can target the pension, encourage everyone to take private pensions (that places the responsibility for their futures onto them) and stress that those not yet aged 45 should not bank on receiving a state pension. Since most people do not want to work forever and the retirement age is increasing it is in their interests to take out a private pension.

If, at the same time, we dismantle regional health authorities to a small administrative core, collapse the number of regional health authorities, the devolvement of responsibility to local levels becomes even more crucial. At this stage we need to advertise our concern and sincerity towards the NHS by publishing a document called *The Health of the Nation* (HMSO, 1993). This will outline our plans to move to a more preventative type of care in order to reduce chronic disease and improve the quality of life. Naturally there will have to be a transfer of funds to cope with that preventative measure and continued investment in acute care. What about those already chronically ill or potentially chronically ill? That is the elderly at-risk group. We have thought of that and are delaying comment until further research is carried out.

Let us consider the consequences, so far, of this obviously fictitious conspiracy:

PROJECT 2000 AND NURSE EMPLOYMENT

Since Project 2000 (P2000) started hospitals have, indeed, developed means of coping without the extra hands on previously experienced by students. The knock-on effect is that those who have replaced the students do not leave (the students did once qualified) which means that there are no vacancies for newly qualified nurses. Indeed, in some areas qualified nurses are taking employment as health care assistants. There is another potential knock-on here: if a manager elects to take on the American model of a qualified nurse per floor (they have responsibility), but a health care assistant is a qualified nurse then there is no reason to employ a qualified nurse. Of course the qualified nurse on lower pay could refuse to take responsibility but the United Kingdom Central Council for Nursing, Midwifery and Health Visiting (UKCC) are looking into ways of passing legislation that will enforce nurses to be accountable, even when off duty. Because regions now need fewer nurses the nursing colleges are being amalgamated, the numbers entering training are being reduced and nurse teachers are being made redundant. The obvious solution would be to place all colleges of nursing into higher education. Unfortunately many universities have realized that they could be taking on an albatross by incorporating colleges of nursing at this stage. Back to the conspiracy: whilst this situation unfolds we embark on a massive advertisement campaign to recruit nurses. It is not a total fallacy because some areas are short of nurses, but advertising convinces people that we are not targetting nurses for the dole.

Consider that you are a newly qualified 21-year-old nurse. Nursing is predominantly a female profession which means, even in these enlightened times, a nurse's role will be secondary to the husband's. You are married and cannot really leave the area. You attend for interview at your trust status hospital to be interviewed by a non-nurse who informs you that he has no vacancies for nurses but could take you on as a level 3 health care assistant. You protest that you are a qualified nurse and receive the retort: okay, sign on the dole. You are not eligible for dole because your husband is earning what is perceived to be a good wage. What would you do, given that you need the money?

Many of the large psychiatric hospitals have closed and a large number of ex-inmates are now wandering the streets, a situation discussed in previous chapters. There have been many problems with ex-psychiatric patients in the UK and in August 1993 the Minister of Health announced that key workers would be appointed for every ex-'mental' patient in the community. It appears that the function of this key worker will be similar to that of the probation officer. A case of keep them on the streets at all costs (or at less cost in this case)?

Then there is the ramifications of the health of the nations. From 1993 there has been talk of charging patients for a GP consultation and charging pensioners for prescriptions. The Health of the Nation Document (HMSO, 1993) identifies five key areas for action: coronary heart disease and strokes, cancers, mental illness, HIV/AIDS and sexual health and accidents. Arguably, the longer we live the more likely we are to suffer from any one or any combination of these. Indeed the document admits that coronary heart disease and strokes are the major causes of ill health and mortality in elderly people; the risk of many types of cancer increases with age; depression, suicide and dementia are more common in the elderly age group; 70% of all fatal home accidents occur in people aged 65 years and over; 300 000 people of 65 and over attend accident and emergency departments every year. There is the odd mention of the aged in these contexts, but generally the elderly are successfully marginalized by this document.

There is talk of: '. . . adding years to life and . . . adding life to years . . .' and yet the main focus is all about reducing deaths in the under–65 age groups. Just a thought but at the time that this document was publicized was that not the retirement age? Is the implication that we can facilitate the deaths of those over 65? The anticipated rise in the over–85 age group is about 34% . . . a potential rise of 34% in the demand for health care and pensions. The debility caused by strokes demands much from the existing resources, hence it makes sense to prevent them. Unfortunately there does appear to be quite a strong genetic link (Black *et al.*, 1984) . . . is this a case for the rise of eugenics? The UK is increasingly moving towards a system where, once the initial problem is eased, we can discharge and informal care is offered by the family and/or volunteers. In these times of health care being economically led being old and ill is an expensive condition. If a charge is levied for GP consultation and hospital beds then it will disadvantage the very groups who need them most. Being chronically ill and old means that your earning power is very limited. The elderly rely, at present, on a pension where every penny counts. Perhaps they could turn off their heating and then they could afford to see the doctor? We are rapidly moving towards the time when Simon and Garfunkel's words are becoming apposite:

God forgive me but an old man without money is pathetique.

The Health of the Nation Document suggests making the best use of resources and the balance of maintaining health . . . not simply health care. What is the best use of these available resources? The document states that if everything is a priority then there is, in effect, no priority (ascribing value to conditions and people again). The emphasis is placed on health rather than care. Emphasis on health places responsibility on the person. During the late 1980s and early 1990s there have been several incidences of patients who have been refused care because of self-inflicted trauma; e.g. one man refused a liver transplant because he was alcoholic, doctors in Manchester refusing to treat smokers for lung conditions

(1993). If the key areas of the Health of the Nation Document are accepted as being preventable then the implication is that each and every person carries some responsibility for their future health. If you smoke, drink, take no exercise or too much exercise then you are putting your health at risk and should not expect others to care for you free of charge.

The UK already charges for ambulance costs when a person is involved in an accident ... presumably because accidents are preventable. Where does this line of argument stop? At those people known to be sexually promiscuous with sexually transmitted diseases? With the uncontrolled diabetic with neuropathy or a leg ulcer? Or at the old man who could not keep himself fit? Shakespeare suggested that we return to childhood: 'sans teeth, sans everything', unfortunately the elderly are not as worthy as children when it comes to receiving health care resources. The success of the Health of the Nation directives will come from:

- **Public policies**: these are already under discussion, make pensioners pay for prescriptions, increase retirement age ... what a shame we cannot find meaningful employment for babies.
- **Healthy surroundings**: in the home and at work; we have all heard of some of the healthy surroundings the elderly experience during winter, it causes hypothermia.
- **Healthy lifestyles**: it may not require money but exercise is irrelevant if you take a poor diet. Recent research suggests that the majority of the elderly population in the UK has a poor diet.
- **High quality health services**: how does this apply to the elderly? There have been horror stories since the mid 1980s that indicate that the elderly are cared for in inappropriate settings and bused out to remote homes miles away from family and friends ... where is the quality? Other cases have illustrated that the elderly are means tested and their property sold to pay for their care.

Age has become expensive because the longer you live the more claims you are likely to make on the state. Acute medicine and surgery are attractive because you can measure the end product; but ageing – you cannot prevent that no matter how effective your preventative medicine is. However, the Health of the Nation Document (HMSO, 1993) does offer some comfort by stressing the importance of monitoring, developing and reviewing the strategy by the Central Health Monitoring Unit. This will carry out a series of epidemiological overviews. Epidemiology is that branch of medical science concerned with the occurrence, transmission and control of epidemic disease. It has come to mean the study of the pattern of any illness. The first study by this unit will be conducted on the elderly, followed by asthma, coronary heart disease and strokes. What's this? The elderly put on a par with disease? It may well mean that the patterns of disease within the elderly population will be studied, but why separate specific diseases? Maybe it is to discover how potentially expensive ageing is. No, this is not cynicism, merely experienced romanticism.

Services for the elderly, along with those for psychiatry and learning difficulties, have always been the marginalized services. Bertrand Russell (1966) once argued that if universal peace could be assured by exterminating the Jews then there would be no reason for not exterminating them; it would be totally ethical. Ethics are devised to support the majority and Russell's argument is based on that which is best for the majority. Morals are more individualistic because they are personally constructed. Ethics can be changed to suit the common good, but whose common good? To refer to Nietzsche (1977) again, all societies are the product of its most powerful people. Ethics can be driven by the need to save money. We should not forget that the Third Reich arose out of economic crisis in prewar Germany. Those who were a burden on the state went to the gas chambers: the deformed, the mentally ill and handicapped and then those who had the wealth, the Jews. Once people have been convinced by ethical arguments they will do anything. Of course not one country in the western world would allow a similar thing to happen in their society.

Earlier in this chapter those people discharged from the large psychiatric hospitals were mentioned. Those people who had no choice but to be prised away from their social arena into an alien world. The hospital, like any institution, has a form of social meaning for the inmates (Reider, 1953; Safirstein, 1967; Geller, 1993). They become psychologically attached to it, just as we do to our 'communities'. To be uprooted and sent to a foreign country is bound to cause separation anxiety. For those people Kundera's (1984) image of being on a tightrope is all the more appropriate. When your roots are pruned away, your safety net dismantled and your only contact with the past is a weekly visitor and a bottle of pills you are very likely to enter into crisis. This may cause you to react violently, in our society it also earns you the right to have a psychiatric probation officer, an entry onto a special supervision register and immediate recall to an institution if you step out of line (various newspapers, 13 August 1993). Did we not used to censor the Russians for similar activities prior to glasnost?

Not content with discharging these people we also collaborate with a process of losing them from the system. Many were placed in the 'landlady scheme': a boarding house where they had to leave the building by 09.30 and could not return before 17.30. Many have no choice other than wandering the streets and seeking shelter wherever they can. Some have been 'expelled' by the landladies for bizarre behaviour and have become the major clientele in various hostels. Their 'key-workers' have lost contact with them and eventually they disappear from the statistics. Consequently the number of 'registered' psychiatric cases reduce and the need to provide a service can be called into question. The Italian experience several years ago achieved this on a national basis, they simply closed the psychiatric hospitals and reported great success; similar reports came from the USA. These reports were false and the problem was merely relocated. The Italian psychiatric population was cared for in shanty towns by informal and untrained carers and the American experience showed little difference (Torrey, 1985). Despite media coverage of the plight of these people in the UK there appears to be very little concern from the majority, except for their own safety. We can allow the creation of psychiatric probation officers because these people are the new under-class. If we do not see them they do not exist. A perception of the majority may be that nothing has really changed because they did not exist when they were contained in large asylums. The setting has merely changed to the 'community'. There is change, however, as there was a form of social meaning in the large hospitals; under house arrest in the community you are much more alone and unable to gain any social meaning.

The experience of a discharged psychiatric inmate could make startling material for a Kafka novel:

Joseph K was guilty. He must be guilty because after they had released him from the hospital, explaining that he was now well, he was being watched. He woke up one morning and was told that he had been placed on a special supervision register. He had no friend to discuss his situation with, they had all been sent elsewhere. K had been discharged from the hospital several months ago. His day to day life had passed by without event until this morning. He had been awoken by a man with the face of an inquisitor, his eyes narrow and his brows thickly knitted. Alongside him was K's landlady her face flushed with concern. K tried to stuff his stained vest into his institutional boxer shorts, his regular sleeping attire from the happy days.

'I'm sorry I woke you,' said the man. 'This community belongs to the majority and whosoever lives here does so with the permission of the majority. You have no such permit, or at least have not produced one.

K was confused, he got out of bed and fumbled in his drawer finding the letter of discharge that he had shown his GP. He handed it to the young man.

'Oh dear, no . . . this will not do . . . see here?' he pointed to the letter head and K nodded, 'this is issued by the hospital that no longer exists; indeed there are some that say it never existed. No, I can't accept this, you need a permit from the majority.'

'How do I get one?' asked K

'You can't just get one,' replied the man, slightly amused.

'He's not like us,' smiled the landlady, 'he doesn't understand.'

'You either have one or you don't,' explained the man. This isn't one . . . do you have another?' K shook his head. He could ask the Charge Nurse at the hospital but the man said it doesn't exist. Should he take a tablet? if he did perhaps the man would go away. 'You haven't? I see.' The man looked, meaningfully, at the landlady and then slowly turned his gaze back to K.

'I could ask at the day centre . . .' he explored.

'The day centre! And pray who could give you a permit there?' sniffed the man.

'Then how am I supposed to get one?'

'He doesn't understand, he's not like us,' said the landlady again.

'Don't adopt that tone with me, Joseph K,' said the man and there was an ironical contempt for K expressed in his gesture. 'I'm your key worker and I'm going to have to place you on a specialist register. You had better behave Joseph K or you'll be taken away.'

The man turned to leave and K received a hard stare from his landlady.

'A word in your ear, Mrs Woman,' said the man, and they left together closing the door firmly behind them.

Joseph K was guilty, he must be, someone had taken his permit to live in the community away.

(Freely adapted from The Castle, Kafka, 1979)

Kafka's novels are studies in normlessness. They generally revolve around characters who suddenly find themselves in a world that makes no sense and where they cannot gain access to the rules. Kafka's examples are works of fiction and yet real examples are being experienced all around us. Lewis (1978) sees three elements to a person's life:

Being alive (biological), leading a life (behavioural) and having a life (quality).

Lewis (1978) stresses that in his opinion having a life is by far the most important in a person's world. We have explored some of these aspects in the earlier chapters but have not concentrated too much on quality of life. Most people living in the 'community' have some semblance of quality in their lives. They have support systems based on friends and relatives. These are things that have developed over time and cannot be created artificially. When that quality is non-existent people can be pushed to extreme actions. Guenter Parche, the man who stabbed tennis player Monica Seles, was described as a loner. Werner, the psychologist who assessed him, reported that the act would never have happened:

. . . if this man had a circle of friends . . .

The depth of the friendship is not really relevant, the networks that we construct serve as anchors and illustrate that we belong, we are connected. This is all part of how we construct social reality. We know where we are placed and where to locate others. We cannot artificially create that for all the people we have thrown out of hospital and forgotten.

The biological concept, being alive, contributes to the quality. A much neglected area is that of disability. The driving force of modern medicine is the acute philosophy. Once we have treated the presenting symptoms as best we can then discharge. Consider that a person's world is constructed through their experience. Their location informs him/her of his/her abilities and it is by way of those abilities that a person relates to the world. You need to get some milk and eggs, so why not get a few other things at the same time. You know where the store is, simply hop into the car, drive down town and there you are. The car won't start, no problem, here comes a bus so you sprint for it and catch it. You are not too happy with having to use a bus because they are dictated by someone else's timetable, not your own, but you can cope until the car is fixed. You can weave in and out of the aisles, avoiding all those slow old people, nip in front of some woman hampered by children and secure a place at the check-out. Nothing really startling or interesting, part of everyday life and something of a background expectancy. Consider the same situation following a stroke. You are a previously fit 40-year old, you go to bed after a good day and suddenly, sometime in the night, your body turns against you. The right side of your brain suffers trauma and the whole left side of your body refuses to work. You still feel okay and are a little bemused by the panic of your family as they rush here and there around you. You are taken to hospital and taught how to walk again, but never as agile as before. You constantly have to position your left arm into a place where it is not cumbersome or damaged. Periodically you convince yourself that you can feel a tingle in your left thumb. Biologically your whole world has turned upside down. You cannot ride a bicycle now ... not that you have for a long time, but you could have last month if you had wanted. You can no longer run, people look at you with the contempt that enforced sympathy brings. The hospital have done their bit, taught you to walk, given you a wheelchair for long hauls until you are used to walking, given you a stick and a list of physiotherapy appointments. You are discharged to your previous life. Remember rehabilitation means to restore to the previous state. Your previous life has gone, a trip to the store for milk and eggs is now a major expedition. Your car is modified but it is now a lifeline ... you can't sprint for a bus if it won't start and the very act of boarding a bus is full of effort. Hodges (1991) reported that hospitals teach you all the wrong things following a stroke, they neglect the new social skills you will need such as asking someone to hold your stick while you board the train. Ordinary people do not know how to approach you, thinking you'll be annoyed if they offer help, so they avoid you ... hence you have to ask.

Being disabled does not mean the quality of your life has totally disappeared but it does mean that practitioners should be aware that it has certainly changed. In the case of the stroke patient a large part of their old life has died and they need guidance about how to come to terms with it. The disabled are a minority group and, as such, tend to have facilities offered as an after-thought; make-shift ramps up stairways that could provoke vertigo in the stoutest of hearts. Often, provision of facilities for the disabled is devolved to local level, and even further to individual businesses. There is little money specifically earmarked for this group. Indeed, many of the services for the disabled are provided by charities.

The final group to be visited in this review of government influence on community health care is the chronically ill. There are many chronic illnesses and these are not confined to the elderly population. The diabetic who is insulin dependent can start with the condition early in life. At the time of writing these people had free prescriptions although there is talk of introducing charges, either directly from the patient or by way of the GP budget. At the current purchasing rate one diabetic can cost, at a conservative estimate, about £500 a year in insulin alone. Then there is the risk of neuropathy which could involve protracted treatment with analgesia and psychotrophic drugs for anything up to 2 years, which could add a further £330 onto the bill each year. That is over £800 a year in drugs alone. Then there is the cost of time spent in consultation.

If GPs are to manage their budgets then people become cost rated. The diabetic becomes unattractive in an economic world. Suppose the day does arrive when he has to pay for his own prescriptions and he is unable to work because of neuropathy. The responsibility is his, and yet the condition is genetic. GPs could be forced into the position of selecting patients on the same basis as insurance companies do in terms of pay out risk. This would make the elderly, the disabled and the chronically ill unattractive and potentially doctorless. At best a system would have to be devised that shared these people out between health centres ... but the elderly population is growing. The link and relationship between economy and health care is growing closer all the time.

There has always been a link between industry and health care. The first health insurance scheme was devised to protect workers prior to the NHS. The scheme only covered the worker, hence illustrating how certain people were valued more than others and how health care has a tradition of targetting those deemed worthy. Health in the work place is a complex issue and provision of services is just as open to abuse as that in the community. Often diseases caused by working conditions have been identified long before they are made recordable. In essence those in power are quite happy to allow workers to perform in conditions that they know will cause life-threatening disease. It is a similar ethical issue to the cannon fodder in wars or the soldiers used to test the effects of radioactive fallout. If it is for the common good then ethically it is okay. Similarly if the majority can receive better benefits by cutting services to minority groups it can only be a good thing.

It is easy to mislead with statistics. Government sources repeatedly issue statements in the UK stating that more is now being spent on the NHS than was spent 20 years ago. This is true in hard cash but not in real terms. Hospitals have closed and patterns of care delivery have been manipulated; people spend less time as inpatients and beds are dismantled. The government spend more to offer a reduced service because of inflation, increases in salaries and expensive drugs being used in preference to, just as effective, cheaper ones. This is a classic example of an institution functioning for itself rather than for the service it is supposed to be delivering.

In the next chapter the ideal community will be compared and contrasted with the real and, hopefully, several of these themes will be drawn together.

REFERENCES

Black, N., Boswell, D., Gray, A. *et al.* (1984) *Health and Disease*, Open University Press, Milton Keynes.

Geller, J.L. (1993) Treating revolving door patients who have hospitalphilia: compassion, coercion and common sense. *Hospital and Community Psychiatry*, 44(2), 141–6.

Gellerman, S. (1974) *Behavioural Science in Management*, Penguin, Harmondsworth, Middlesex.

HMSO (1989) *Working for Patients*, HMSO, London.

HMSO (1993) *The Health of the Nation*, HMSO, London.

Hodges, B.E. (1991) Participant observations of rehabilitation. Unpublished.

Kafka, F. (1979) *The Castle*, Penguin, Harmondsworth, Middlesex.

Kundera, M. (1984) *The Unbearable Lightness of Being*. Faber and Faber, London.

Lewis, C.S. (1978) *The Abolition of Man*, Fount, London.

Marx, K. (1955) *Selected Works*, Foreign Languages Publishing House, Moscow.

Nietzsche, F. (1977) *A Nietzsche Reader*, Penguin, Harmondsworth, Middlesex.

Reider, N. (1953) A Type of Transference to Institutions. *Bulletin of the Menninges Clinic*, 17, 58–63.

Russell, B. (1966) *Philosophical Essays*, Allen and Unwin, London.

Safirstein, S.L. (1967) Institutional transference. *Psychiatry Quarterly*, 41, 557–66.

Torrey, E.F. (1985) *Surviving Schizophrenia*, Harper and Row, London.

Weber, M. (1949) *The Methodology of the Social Sciences*, Free Press, New York.

CHAPTER 6

The city at night

In order to paint the other side of an otherwise idyllic city, Heller (1970) has his hero Yosarian walk around the city at night. Here he witnesses the darker side of life. In similar vein the movie director David Lynch (1986) utilizes this genre for his film *Blue Velvet*. The message is that most of us let our lives pass by in a rosy hue. We safeguard the security and close our eyes to anything that might threaten that. Lynch utilizes pastel colours for the idealized life and darkness for 'reality'. This style has been adopted for the last chapter in this section.

THE IDEAL WORLD

In an ideal world there would be no −isms and everyone would be equal. In this world community would welcome and care for its natives and generally add to the quality of life. Lewis (1990) suggests that it is for biologists and philosophers to discuss what life is and that the rest of us have the less ambitious task of examining what people mean by the word life. Lewis is mistaken if he truly believes that this is a less ambitious task. Again in the UK there are possibly 57 million different definitions of life. Life can be described as something an organism loses at death but it is far more than that. A person's life is his/hers just as much as his or her nose is. It is unique and special. In an ideal world the community acknowledges this and functions purely for the good of the residents. Community, then, as a title conveys various meanings. In Lawrence's (1975) sense it suggests:

. . . life itself, warmth.

In Chapter 1 this sentiment is echoed by suggesting that if a person feels that he belongs in a particular location then that is his community.

Belonging stimulates a feeling of connectedness and warmth. It is one of the ideals of life. Community also suggests connectedness, that is groups of people with a common bond, be it kinship or tribal ties. Being connected in this way means that we can rely on our neighbours for help in times of crisis. Robb (1954) described Bethnal Greeners and stated that their immobility ensured that they were surrounded by people like themselves. People know how their neighbours expect them to behave and the likely effects of their behaviour on others; they know what will happen if they go outside the norms that direct behaviour. Robb (1954) is illustrating the predictability of community life. Durant (1959) defined community as '. . . a territorial group of people with a common mode of living striving for common objectives . . .'. Frankenberg (1975) suggests that social networks are composed of groups and categories. The group has common aims which impose a group boundary (inclusivity and exclusivity) and carries the implication of social interaction between the individuals comprising it. The category means a collection of people who share certain characteristics but do not necessarily interact with each other (men and women are examples of categories). Hence, in Frankenberg's sense all groups are partial categories but not all categories are groups. Friendship is a category in that a person's friends have in common the fact that they interact with the person but not necessarily with each other (Frankenberg, 1975). The individual may view the structure of his community much more matter of factly:

> There are mates, friends and acquaintances. Mates you do anything for, you give them anything they want . . . Friends you lend but don't give . . . Acquaintances you don't want to know . . .
> (Morris and Morris, 1963)

Relationships in any community are reciprocal. In the above passage mates are people you do anything for and in return they give you anything. This notion has been a theme of previous chapters and was reinforced by Skidmore's (1986) findings. Friendships are the expressed expectations of our own ideals. Similarly the world becomes the ideal that we express. Consequently, then, as in friendship when most people are loathe to test the relationship, the world is built on a collection of ideals that are rarely tested.

One extreme is the notion that there is an after life and this offers a person a security about living. Similarly if there is a higher intelligence directing all things we need not worry about anything that happens, it is the will of the Great One. This notion has permeated much of everyday life to the extent that most things have become background expectancies (things that we generally agree exist but rarely question). Consider love: it makes the world go around and binds people together but there is no objective way of measuring the emotion. However, most of us know that it exists and we have timetabled events to reinforce its existence – St Valentine's Day. Our emotions are placed on a continuum so that we can categorize those people we are located with. We may love a few, feel various forms of affection for many, hate a few, dislike many and be totally indifferent to the majority. To locate people even further and construct our community with greater solidity we can subcategorize love: sexual love, parental love, sibling love and so on. These titles do not so much advertise to the world where these people are located, but identify to the individual where they are placed with regard to each other. Once located we can negotiate roles and expectations just like the mate, friend and acquaintance model.

So far, then, it has been suggested that a person's community is based on: predictability, connectedness, groups and categories, and ideals (e.g. love). As we look out at our world all these things help us to make sense of that world. Our community is an area that helps us to break down the world into smaller and meaningful shapes. Chermayeff and Tzonis (1971) argue that community '. . . as an idea and fact has been extended . . . to an immeasurably greater spectrum of human contacts than ever before in history . . .'. They are alluding to the global village here and suggest that the growth in urban society has destroyed the possibility of man's identification with familiar places. It could be argued that they severely underestimate man. It has been suggested in previous chapters that man functions on two levels: the public and the private. The identification of familiar places arises from the private and, essentially, idealized world. Hence, whereas the idea and fact of community may have extended the ideal and actual community is fairly static.

Ideally what does each person get out of his community? In a sense each person views his/her community as a similar image to many communities. Each community makes up a society (or village) and that collection of societies constructs the world. Consequently that which can be expected from the community is replicated in the world. The community cares about its members and because it cares there is security and support by just living there. Because each member knows that it exists s/he does not need to test it. This feeling of being cared for helps the members to gain confidence to explore the world outside the community, because there is always somewhere to return to. Each expedition into the world is accompanied by the norms of the community. In other words because the community is a product of the individual then each individual carries their community with them into the wider world. This permits the Lippman syndrome to occur (to define and then see). Thus a person will enter each new area anticipating many things and then selectively collecting data that confirms the preconceived views. The person looking for evidence of love will find it on buses, trains, in the streets and the parks. The person looking for evidence of lust will find it in identical places at the same point in time. It is merely a question of interpretation.

Community can be analogous with places of interest and beauty spots. There are prominent features in most countries that tourists flock to see but one cannot describe the country through these. The features of a person's community are those that we have discussed above and about these there will be consensus of agreement between groups and categories. A person's community consists of lovers, friends, families, mates and acquaintances. Each person, group or category offers a sense of meaning to the person. Communities cannot exist if people do not feel that they belong. In this sense, then, the measure of community is on the emotional level and not merely a matter of fact. Measuring how many people live in a 3-mile radius, how many are blood relatives, or how many interact with the same people does not describe the community. Because it is based on caring the community looks after its members or, when ill equipped to do so, brings in agents to care. Initially we subscribe to this caring ethos through our taxes so that our community can be serviced by hospitals and schools. On a similar economic level we pay local taxes and elect local councillors to administer the economy on our behalf to improve social conditions for the community. We trust that there is a shared pride and mutual concern in our community. Some communities band together at certain times to advertise their connectedness: the village fête, best kept garden contest, street parties and processions. The common goal theory suggests that people are bound together by shared motives (Sherif, 1966). The motive for community is one of mutual caring and any activity shared can be seen to reinforce this.

Consequently in the ideal community people will watch out for each other. There will be special places of succour for the less advantaged and specialist centres for those needing help. Generally it is everybodies' right to receive care. Those out of work will receive financial help from the state; the elderly frail will receive material support in the shape of meals on wheels and periodic visits from health care staff. Children receive equal educational opportunities, regardless of their background. In this respect mankind has retrospectively reconstructed his world. The existentialist atheists (Sartre, 1948; Heidegger, 1977) argue that man first of all exists, encounters himself, surges up in the world and defines himself afterwards. Furthermore, man is nothing more than that which he makes of himself (Sartre, 1948). The existentialist view is that man's negotiation with the world is, in fact, the act of fashioning mankind: '. . . I am creating a certain image of man as I would have him be' (Sartre, 1948). This of course presents us with a problem since if God does not exist then everything would be permitted (Dostoyevsky, 1966). This places man in the situation of, as Sartre (1948) states, being condemned to freedom if man had not constructed his social meaning with such rigour. The 'community spirit' is an extension of that which God stands for. It offers a meaning to existence and liberates us from being condemned to freedom. Marx (1955) has argued that if God did not exist man would have to invent him. Similarly if community did not exist man would have to invent it; and the same of love and friendship.

Descartes (1968) stated: 'Conquer yourself rather than the world'. Within this argument man creating his own world is the same thing. A combination of Nietzsche and Sartre would develop the argument that community is created by the enforcement of the ideals of that society's great (most powerful) men and this then becomes the truth of man. In reality, things will be such as men have decided that they should be. Thus this idealistic, caring community has been created by our agents for the common good from their own altruistic thoughts. These thoughts are merely a reflection of those that we all share. After all the community is an extension of the family and all that it stands for to a larger scale. In Laing's (1971) words: 'To be in the same family is to feel the same "family" inside'. Similarly to be in the community is to feel that community inside. It has been suggested, above, that community is more a feeling than a measurable structure. Hegel (1977) suggests that the world is 'a unity of the given and the constructed'. The given is locked in tradition and the constructed are those landmarks that produce a consensus of agreement within groups and categories. The consensus of agreement is that there is goodness in community and that care in and by the community is better for everyone. In similar vein the picture postcards we receive from friends when they visit new places offers an idyllic view of cities and countries. Naturally the blackspots are not highlighted by the tourist board. In addition, as we have explored in Chapter 4, the tourist has not got the time to explore new places effectively and sticks to the landmarks and beauty spots. His experience of the country is one-sided and idealized and we will pick up that perception of the country from his accounts. Similarly the accounts we will receive from our relatives about the place we live in will be idealized.

CANDID CAMERA

Community, arguably, provides support and care for its natives. That includes all the services from education, health care and prisons. The motive is to protect its members be they sick or under threat. When we catch a glimpse of what reality is really like we tend to suppress it or redefine it. Lewis (1971) argues that this is how we respond to criminals:

> . . . the criminal ceases to be a person, a subject of rights and duties, and becomes merely an object on which society can work . . .

He goes on to argue that this is exactly how Hitler treated the Jews and that they were objects; not killed for ill desert but because, by his theory, they were a disease in society. Lewis (1971) presents an argument congruent with that outlined above for the fluidity of ethics. If society can make and remake man at its pleasure, its pleasure may be humane or homicidal. Either way, argues Lewis, rulers have become owners. These rulers are, of course, our elected representative. Lewis goes on to argue that if religion became inconvenient to the Government, it has already been labelled a neurosis by some schools of psychology and, as such, those practicing religion could be subjected to a compulsory cure.

Lewis feels that there would be little resistance to such moves because two world wars have necessitated vast curtailments of liberty to the extent that we have grown accustomed to our chains. This enslavement has occurred so gradually that we are unaware of it. Furthermore, in line with the argument proffered above, Lewis feels that the increasing complexity and precariousness of our economic life have forced Government to take over many of the spheres of activity once left to choice or chance. Consequently the modern state exists to do us good or make us good.

Making us good is that which happens to the deviants, doing us good is that to which the rest of us are subjected. A stroll around our city at night will reveal many horrors about which we may not care to recognize. We are on the brink of accepting that certain minority groups are mere objects and as such are devoid of rights. The plight of the long-term mentally ill has been explored and the prospects for the elderly used as a theme. The implications of deconstructing the welfare state, however, have serious implications for the survival of 'community'. The very structure and meaning of the welfare state is under threat. Benefits are to come under close scrutiny, student grants are already under threat in the UK. We are given parallels that exist in the rest of Europe and in the USA. However, the ethic of our society is that anyone in employment, certainly from 1950, has been contributing for:

1. A health care system which offers care from the cradle to the grave for him and his family.
2. A state pension at the age of 65.
3. Certain benefits during hard times, such as unemployment benefit and child allowances.

The knowledge of the things that he has been contributing for have added to the comfort he derives from belonging to a community. Since the mid 1980s there has been a deconstruction of those things. In terms of health care the Government has moved to an increasingly privatized model. This system, we are informed, works very well in other parts of Europe and the USA, however the natives of those countries do not have to pay twice, i.e. to the state and to an insurance company for the same service. Similarly, many people were convinced that the National Insurance scheme would be an investment for the future in the shape of a state pension. Noises are now being made that suggests the contrary. Would be pensioners could, in fact, end up paying into two systems: National Insurance which maintains the welfare state and a private pension scheme.

However, no person really gains a glimpse of what the real community is like until they experience it. For example, when a close relative, such as a parent or spouse, is taken ill and they realize that their investment in the health care system does not guarantee treatment, they hit upon waiting lists or lack of resources. Alternatively their elderly relative receives acute treatment for a stroke and is discharged to the care of a single parent, working son. This is one aspect of the reality of community care. The institutional side of care has been carried out, it is now the problem of the relatives. The son will be dangled the carrot of the possibility of sheltered accommodation but in the short term he must make do. He has to negotiate time off work and care for a mother who previously cared for him. His mother will have to bear the indignity of being toiletted by her son and he will need to gather all his forbearance to cope with role-reversal. When he tries to explain his experience to another they will only gather a perception (Buber, 1970) of that experience and will reconstruct the events as he explains them.

Each experience is unique; it cannot be successfully conveyed to another. In addition only one-third of the population will experience the 'severe' aspects of health care and, consequently, belong to the minority. Society's view of minorities has been reviewed previously. A third of the population is a rather large minority, one might argue. Certainly but then the third is subgrouped into the mentally ill, learning difficulties, chronic disease, acute disease and elderly care. Each of these will have a value in terms of being invested with personship; in short some will be more of a minority than others. If some of these subgroups can be successfully marginalized then they are lost from the figures and the total category is reduced. Normalization is a structured way of marginalizing a group. The suggestion is that the group no longer exists because they have been integrated into the normal population, hence there is no need for a specialist service.

If we consider people with learning difficulties many persons within this group look different. Many people react to that which they see. When people look different from the majority they are immediately treated with segregation. People with different skin colours are subjected to prejudice and they have effective powers of communication. What chance, then, has a person who looks different and fails to communicate effectively? It is not that long ago that there was a lobby in the UK and the USA to have these people sterilized. They were in danger of losing their rights as a person whilst, at the same time, being normalized. If we accept the principle of normalization, that is that it is based on caring, it is almost as though we have two forces pulling in opposite directions. In Tonnies' (1955) terms we have Gemeinschaft (community, a term embodying relationships, caring and love) representing normalization pulling against Gesellschaft (society, a term representing mechanical, public and society). This theme is quite apposite since the two terms are synonymous with public (Gesellschaft) and private (Gemeinschaft). Gesellschaft has become the origin and expression of public opinion and tendencies and is not really representative of the people. Tonnies (1955) states that:

One goes into Gesellschaft as one goes into a strange country.

In reality, however, there is no such opposition since both actions (to sterilize and to normalize) are both tools of Gesellschaft. They are not offered with any feeling of community but represent the desire of society. The assumption is that by sterilizing the deviant it will reduce the population of future deviants; we know this to be false. The expressed intention of normalization is that the child with learning difficulties has a better chance of being integrated into society by this mode; evidence suggests that this is also false. McCauley *et al.* (1994) illustrate that adolescents who experienced the special school had far better 'career' prospects than a matched sample who experienced the 'normalizing' process. In addition the services offered for learning difficulties in the main stream school were subject to abuse by both teachers and pupils. The remedial class, for example, was often used as a punishment for troublesome pupils. In addition, because the service was no longer entitled, 'special' teachers without specialist training were expected to deal with pupils who had learning difficulties. At the end of the 4-year study McCauley *et al.* (1994) found that all of the subjects from the special school had obtained full-time employment, albeit menial, whereas only one subject from the main stream system had secured any type of employment, and that was a YTS scheme.

The specialist system may well separate a person from the wider society but it is at least focused on that person. It considers their rights, needs and obligations rather than how they should be trained to mimic the wider population. The specialist system offers them the opportunity to develop the skills that will enable them to improve the quality of their lives, a point echoed by Hodges (1991) in preceding chapters. Placing a person with learning difficulties within main stream education exposes them to the competitive element that educationalists have battled with for decades. Furthermore it exposes them to a competitive system where they lack the skills to compete equally. The principle that underpins normalization is noble, but demands the resources to carry it through. Resources make demands on the economy, which we have agreed is finite. This situation is identical to that of the long-term mentally ill. The principle of placing them in the community is noble, but demands the resources to be anything like successful. This argument is logical to most people, for anything to work it must have the necessary equipment otherwise it is doomed to fail. Without the provision of the necessary equipment there has to be other motives for implementation. Those motives can only be to transfer responsibility and save money; a Gesellschaft (society) motive rather than one that has concern for people.

It has already been suggested that society represents the common opinion, the desire of the majority. Seymour (1993), using the Bosnian war victims as an exemplar, asks whether or not Britain cares anymore.

Our society, he argues, was famed for caring about the suffering of others and for over a century spearheaded the supply of aid to impoverished nations. He identifies the past decade as having illustrated an unpleasant change when Britain has had:

> ... governments which put compassion well down their list of priorities ...

Seymour (1993) states that he hoped that this was not a reflection of the heart and spirit of the people and yet surveys indicate that less than 30% supported the provision of medical aid to Bosnia. He concludes by arguing that failing to save these victims will not save our health service. In a truly caring world Seymour is perfectly correct. There are indeed thousands of families who would not be alive today had the UK not given them residency. Much of that aid, however, was given when the UK was economically well placed. Over the years we have become willing slaves of the welfare state (Lewis, 1971) whereby we support the policies of our leaders because it will be of ultimate benefit. In many ways each person has become detached from community in Tonnies' (1955) sense by the rapid rise of society. It has been argued in Chapters 1 and 2 that the move from the rural community offered the opportunity for more people to become 'privatized'; that is to realize larger portions of their private world. The consequence of this is that a person becomes more insular and is more willing to allow others to organize. As Lewis (1971) states:

> What assurances have we that our masters will or can keep the promise which induced us to sell ourselves? Let us not be deceived about "Man taking charge of his own destiny". All that can really happen is that some men will take charge of the destiny of the others ... The more completely we are planned the more powerful they will be.

The above was originally written in 1958 when the welfare state was in full swing and the affluent worker was on the rise (Lockwood, 1958). Lewis would no doubt be horrified by the accuracy of his concerns today. The rise of the affluent worker can be seen as a benchmark for the demise of the caring community. It provided the workers with money and ultimately alienated them from their solidarity as workers. Their lives, in short, became dominated by economic freedom. The consequence of this was that they moved away from their working class communities (Skidmore, 1986). The mid 1980s witnessed the onset of a terminal condition in the trade union movement. It could be argued that once the generation who had helped construct the movement out of common suffering retired there was little to hold it together. The new generation had been born into affluence and could only gain a perception of the history that created their affluence.

Working men and women comprise the largest majority of the population. Their party had been one of socialism, basically equal rights for all, fair pay and a caring society. The Conservative party have been vindicated in their view of society by staying in power since it is quite obvious that the natives do not desire that type of society. Even the Labour party is having to distance itself from its socialist principles in order to survive. The willing slaves are endorsing the ideals of their leaders.

The Cambridge marxists (Blunt, Burgess and McClean) along with other intellectuals of the late 1920s and 1930s claim that they were turned to communism after witnessing the suffering of the Jarrow marchers (Philby, 1968). Similarly the socialist movement grew from suffering. Many working men joined the communist party because there was no real alternative for the working man. When the socialist movement started, led by Keir Hardie, they joined in droves. The movement was seen to be so threatening for the government of the day that many of the leaders of the movement, notably Hardie, were imprisoned for treason. The history of the Trade Union movement and the Labour Party is etched with strife and suffering, from the Tolpuddle Martyrs to the miners. Suffering becomes less of an impact within a privatized society and we are in danger of moving full circle. There is nothing like experiencing suffering or witnessing suffering to recognize how powerless we are to prevent it.

In times past attempts were made to solve the social problems by policy. The workhouse, for example, was seen to be a bold, ruthless and successful attempt to solve pauperism (Longmate, 1974). The poor fell into two groups: those unable to maintain themselves such as the old, very young, the sick, crippled, blind and the insane; and those who merely lacked work. Sound familiar? This notion of returning to the past will be further explored in Part Two. Briefly, the workhouse was seen as a solution to a problem of economy. In some parishes, once the workhouse was opened the weekly pension for the poor was terminated. In some cases, where some 150 paupers were registered for the pension, the workhouse residency never rose above 30 (Longmate, 1974). Longmate (1974) reveals the writing of a 1727 man: 'A workhouse is a name that carries along with it the idea of correction and punishment ... our poor have taken such an aversion to living in it.' One should remember that the Poor Law dictated that workhouses should provide conditions that were less desirable than those outside. Consequently we return to the theme of this chapter that those viewed as a burden upon society eventually lose their rights and obligations. Society can do to them for their own good, regardless of their wishes.

The workhouse philosophy placed the responsibility for being ill back in the hands of the sufferer and their relatives. Simultaneously it had the effect of reducing the registered poor by losing them in the system.

Looking around our cities at night reveals evidence of similar philosophies.

This section has strived to provide an almost philosophical background against which the concept of caring in and by the community can be examined. In Part Two the concepts of care and caring will be explored through the motif of the family.

REFERENCES

Buber, M. (1970) *I and Thou*, T. and T. Clark, Edinburgh.
Chermayeff, S. and Tzonis, A. (1971) *Shape of Community: realization of human potential*, Penguin, Harmondsworth, Middlesex.
Descartes, R. (1968) *Discourse on Method and the Meditations*, Penguin, Harmondsworth, Middlesex.
Dostoyevsky, F. (1968) *Crime and Punishment*, Penguin, Harmondsworth, Middlesex.
Durant, R. (1959) *Watling: a survey of social life on a new housing estate*, King, London.
Frankenberg, R. (1975) *Communities in Britain*, Penguin, Harmondsworth, Middlesex.
Hegel, G.W.F. (1977) *Phenomenology of Spirit*, Oxford University Press, Oxford.
Heidegger, M. (1977) *The Question Concerning Technology and Other Essays*, Colophon, London.
Heller, J. (1970) *Catch 22*, Cape, London.
Laing, R.D. (1971) *Self and Others*, Penguin, Harmondsworth, Middlesex.
Lawrence, D.H. (1975) *Sons and Lovers*, Penguin, Harmondsworth, Middlesex.
Lewis, C.S. (1971) *Undeceptions*, Bles, London.
Lewis, C.S. (1990) *Studies in Words*, Cambridge University Press, Cambridge.
Lockwood, D. (1958) *The Blackcoated Worker*, Allen and Unwin, London.
Longmate, N. (1974) *The Workhouse*, Temple Smith, London.
Lynch, D. (1986) *Blue Velvet*, CBS/Fox.
McCauley, P. *et al.* (1994) *Normalisation or Neglect* (to be published).
Marx, K. (1955) *Selected Works*, Foreign Languages Publishing House, Moscow.
Morris, T. and Morris, P. (1963) *Pentonville: a sociological study of an English prison*, Routledge and Kegan Paul, London.
Philby, K. (1968) *My Silent War*, Grove Press, New York.
Robb, J.H. (1954) *Working Class Anti-semite*, Tavistock, London.
Sartre, J.P. (1948) *Existentialism and Humanism*, Methuen, London.
Seymour, D. (1993) Does Britain care anymore? *Daily Mirror*, 17 August, p. 8.
Sherif, M. (1966) *Group Conflict and Cooperation: their social psychology*, Houghton Miffin, New York.
Skidmore, D. (1986) The sociology of friendship. University of Keele, PhD Thesis.
Tonnies, F. (1955) *Community and Association*, Routledge and Kegan Paul, New Fetter Lane, London.

Care and Caring

CHAPTER 7

A kingdom of families

Part One painted a rather grim picture of a person's geography, it is hoped that this section will balance the picture to some degree. In the previous section geography was used as a theme, this section utilizes the family for reasons which should become apparent.

FAMILY

The family is the basic unit of caring in our society. There are policies and laws that enforce the idealistic notions of the family. Families have been subjected to study for many years (Wilmot, 1963; Goode, 1964) and each study has struggled to develop a meaningful definition. It could be argued that, like community, a definition is unhelpful and that family exists for those members who feel they belong. However, there is a concept, or expectancy, of what a normal family should be. It is against this idealized notion, which is much clearer than the ideal community, that a person compares his own experience. Being the basic communal group the family has been a rich source of media attention, both fact and fiction. To a large degree the family is an institution: it has history, tradition, process and power (Bilton *et al.*, 1987). Tonnies (1955) refers to family as the gemeinschaft of blood (see Chapter 6) and that it denotes unity of being. He argues that it represents the truly human and supreme form of community. In a simplistic sense Tonnies appears to view community as comprising three elements: kinship, neighbourhood and friendship; all noble and caring relationships. Initially this text is concerned only with the first element, kinship.

Every person belongs to a country (Part One) and within that country he/she builds his/her castle – the home. Tonnies (1955) argues that this home constitutes a realm wherein the body of kinship is likewise constituted. People reside in the home under one protecting roof, share possessions and pleasures, sit and feed at the same table. The single protecting roof is symbolic in that the spirit of the family extends beyond the walls of the home. Just as a person carries his country with him (Part One) so too does the family member carry the family with him. Tonnies (1955) suggests that the average human being feels best and is most cheerful if he is surrounded by his family. Tonnies uses the term in an extended sense to include close blood relatives. In modern times we have reduced the meaning to encompass the couple living together in a sexual relationship. Most studies agree that the cornerstone of the family is mutual love and affection. Laing (1971) locates the study of the family very succinctly:

> We speak of families as though we all know what families are . . . The more one studies family dynamics, the more unclear one becomes . . .

The strength of Laing's statement lies in the first sentence since there is a consensus of agreement about what a family is. Whether or not we belong to a family we feel that we 'know' what is meant by a family. In this sense the family is an ideal type in the same sense that sociologists create 'ideal types' in order to set up a series of categories or continuums. The ideal type allows distinctions of transition to be made, such as Tonnies' (1955) community to society, or Weber's (1949) traditional to legal-rational authority, or Durkheim's (1964) mechanical to organic solidarity. With regard to the family it allows us to place the blame for all social problems on the dysfunctive family. Bell (1956) suggests that the 'romantic notion of the past that sees society as having once been made up of small "organic", close knit communities that were shattered by industrialism . . .' lies beyond the theory of social disorganization.

The 'ideal' family has been used in this way to illustrate the break down of society (Part One). Initially viewed in the extended sense, as Tonnies uses the term, the transition from extended to nuclear family was felt to be a threat to society. It is crucial to disseminate the differences between the close knit family (i.e. parents and children) and the blood ties of the extended family. It could be argued that the family has always been nuclear and the networking involved with an extended family was instrumental a process of exchange, baby sitting for instance). Bell (1956) suggests that improvements in transport and communications have brought men into closer contact with each other and bound them in new ways. Hence the functions of the extended family have been taken over by new networks (friends and neighbours). The basic unit, however, is the family and that ideal type is central to all else whether we experience a family or not. Laing (1971) argues that

> The child is born into a family which is the product of the operations of human beings already in this world.

The ideal family is still viewed as two parents and their offspring. All members love and care for each other. More importantly the family is where we gain our first experience and knowledge of role. It offers us the framework for all our social interactions. Gender roles are shaped by the family and the traditional division of labour is still perpetrated by the media. The ideal family has a clear breadwinner role (male) and a complementary role (female); the breadwinner provides and the 'complementaree' cares. Naturally, it is much more complex than this because the child who is born into the family (or its substitute) develops much of how he should relate to the world through his experience of the family. That is: how one should behave within a gender role, which emotions can be expressed and which cannot, that identity for the male arises from what one does. Unfortunately it also perpetrates the continuation of stereotypical behaviour. All these things are points of agreement in the majority of families. Consequently when one ventures from the family they carry the norms of the family with them and indulge in the Lippman syndrome (define then see). It is a short step, then, from making the connection that other families are like one's own, broadly speaking. There will be differences, such as more or less affection, but the general principles will be adhered to.

Carrying the tenets of the family with us in our everyday encounters allows connections to be made with a wider society. In Part One the importance of predictability was emphasized at a personal level. This is equally true of groups. The values shared by a group when recognized in other groups offer a sense of connectedness with a wider society. If others are like us then the world is a safer place. Laing (1971) argues that the 'family' is transfered to other groups within which an individual interacts. Thus, just as the family becomes a medium by which to link its members (Laing, 1971), so too does it become a medium by which individuals can link groups – a sense of community. Family members, then, have an invested interest in preserving the family, for not to do so would threaten their very world. Parker (1976) suggests that the family is society's primary agent of socialization. To this one would add that it is the primary source of cementing the meaning of society.

The home is the place where many leisure activities take place and this also helps form the framework for how one 'plays' outside the home. Play is an essential part of the support process in that it allows relaxed interaction in a structured way. Most animals learn interactive skills through play (Lorenz, 1967) and humans are no different. Play allows the offspring of a family to interact with a wider society in a less than formal way. That is not to say that play does not have formal rules, only that the consequences of the outcomes are less severe than in a real situation. Many adults use drunkeness in a similar way: 'I must be excused . . . I was drunk and didn't know what I was doing' is similar to 'It was only a game . . .'. The natural consequence of this is that children learn on two levels: the public level where they play the game of life and abide by the rules, and the private level where they can try and do as they will and blame it on play when caught. Play also assists physical contact and through play we learn which contact is pleasurable and which undesirable. Play within the context of the family is safe.

The family, then, is important to its members because it normally provides a secure emotional base which buffers the stresses encountered when participating in society. For many members it will be an extension, albeit modified, of the private world. The reality of the family will be strengthened by its own timetable that revolves around its members. Monday to Friday being work and school days may mean the home is vacated for most of the day. Evenings will be devoted to feeding, some house cleaning and relaxation and preparation for the next day. Weekends will involve the members in family activities which cement the bonds between them. The ritual of family life reinforces the notions of mutual caring and of the family being part of the member. Consequently if a member of the family is hurt, the whole of the family is hurt. We will return to this aspect when considering dysfunction later in this chapter.

NEIGHBOURS

The links that a family makes with immediate society are likely to be with those who live in close proximity, what have become known as neighbours. The term is used, post-industrially, as a term of reference to locate groups and/or individuals in relation to others. It does not convey the same meaning that it held in the 1950s for example. Prior to the affluent worker neighbours were more than people who lived nearby. Other than geographical location they also would be connected through occupation. Hence there existed aspects of everyday living that was shared. Men would travel to work together and share their leisure time; they would have common associates and friends. Women would pass the time of day together, linked through the men folk, share childminding and even work together in part-time jobs. The 'working class' community of the 1950s was linked and bonded in several ways that facilitated solidarity. Whole streets would often take an annual holiday or day trip together, thus advertising inclusivity. All the industry in one town would close for the summer holiday and this facilitated the community spirit. Holiday spots were traditional and influenced by family economy (usually the nearest coastal resort which the family had knowledge of and, thus, could gauge the likely expense). Because they were traditional the chances were that you would meet someone from the same town whilst on holiday. This further facilitated the view that one belonged to a community.

With regard to work, many sons would follow their fathers into a certain line of work. This was very common in mining communities. Consequently both father and son became located through similar people and possibly even share work colleagues. In the South Yorkshire coal fields sons even inherited their father's first name or nickname (Skidmore, 1986). The effect is to locate a person even more within a certain group. Knowledge of a person's ancestors implies knowing a person's history. Frankenberg (1975) points out that:

> ... to be a miner in Ashton is to be in the swim and share the life-experience not only of the majority but also of the group which almost completely dominates social life.

The weekly social life of the working classes was also fairly structured with the prominence of the working man's club. These were liberally scattered across the working class communities and would often be a gathering point for annual holidays, in some cases they would be the administrative centre. The social construction of the community was fairly secure in the 1950s because most working class homes evolved around the place of work and were village like in structure. The small communities were safe from the diluting effect of major towns. Indeed the trip to town would be a weekly trip for market day (Chapters 1 and 2).

The village structure, limited wages (remember that there was no sick pay scheme for many working men for a good part of the 1950s) and connectedness in various ways (work and through marriage) fostered the concept of neighbourliness. The rise of the affluent worker changed that structure irrevocably. Frankenberg (1975) describes how the miner did not save extra cash but spent it on leisure. There was no real incentive to save. Should a new piece of furniture be needed he would work harder for a few weeks. This was fostered by the precarious nature of the job, the budgeting of a limited wage and rises and falls in earnings. However, as the 1950s drew to an end the notion of the standard wage came in, along with sick pay and holiday pay. People suddenly had the wherewithal to buy their own property and move away from the 'village'. They were encouraged to take this step by improvement in transport and, eventually, the buying power of their wages to enter into loans in order to buy their own motor car. The consequence of these changes was to erode the notion of the neighbour. People became connected only through work and all the social reinforcement rituals disappeared.

> ... individuals have grown more estranged from one another. The old primary group ties of family and local community have been shattered; ancient parochial faiths are questioned ... As a result ... relations between individuals are tangential and compartmentalized rather than organic ...

> Bell, 1956

Bell (1956) goes on to argue that because of the move to a mass society the individual loses a coherent sense of self. In fact this has not happened because the individual has been able to construct a reality based on his ideals because of the opportunity to become more privatized. The extended family and the link with neighbours through work may have disappeared but now he can construct networks based on friendship.

These can be maintained by improved communication networks and need not be put to the test since they are not local. In this sense a person is protecting his image of 'community'. The nuclear family is still very much the home base offering the same functions. Neighbours, however, have become people who live close by with no other connection except spatial sharing. In some communities immediate neighbours never communicate (Rope, 1969). The fact that the fears of social disorganization have never been realized is indicative of man's need to feel that he belongs and is located. Where structures do not exist he will create them. To reiterate, from Part One, if community did not exist man would create it.

In short, then, the idealized organic folk community (gemeinschaft) is alive and well and living in the private world of the self. Indeed, prominent members of the 'new villages' (urban overspills) often strive to revive the village spirit by organizing village fêtes, morris dancing and barn dances. Unfortunately the community spirit cannot be artificially created. The 'industrial' village was bonded in several ways: through economy, occupation, marriage ties and blood links; it had shared timetables, rituals and social events; in addition there was a sense of isolation from the major town. Many of these villages have been surrounded by urban development and have become the new, cul-de-sac, urban overspill villages, often due to their quaintness. They are, however, no longer linked to a local industry and the natives could work hundreds of miles apart in totally unconnected jobs. The opportunity, then, does not exist for developing common timetables. So, in a material sense the community does not exist as it did. In a spiritual sense, because the natives will it, it exists as a feeling.

The same process of projecting the family onto neighbouring groups will continue and neighbours will rally round during a crisis. Friendships may even form in the locality. Friendships in post-industrial 'communities' reinforce the idealistic notion of friendship more, since they are relationships of choice. There are no kinship ties or workplace commonalities to bond the relationship. The implication is that people enter into friendships because they find each other attractive, hence offering a sense of worth to each partner. He is my friend because he likes me, rather than we are friends because we work together. In the construction of social meaning these networks will be stronger, on a spiritual (organic) level than during the romanticized 'communities'. The fact that they belong to the private world and will never be tested (see Part One) is not relevant. A person's world is real in the way he constructs it. The family is real in the sense of shared consensus of agreement based on each member's private world, and networks are an extension of the family, that which each member carries with them. For this reason the mass society is not likely to occur in the sense that Bramson (1961) believed it would.

THE INFLUENCE OF CHANGE

It has been suggested in the previous section that the traditional view of the past 'community' life is romanticized. The belief in the structure of community life, however, offered security for all members of society. When changes are recognized the intellectuals of any society attempt to explain the consequences by way of ideal types. This is normally based on what society will lose rather than what will be gained or preserved. Man has a self-interest in maintaining the predictability of his world and, consequently, will uphold his ideals or retrospectively reconstruct the past to make sense of it. Weber (1949) argues that all actions are rational, certainly they are in retrospect. We have not, as a society, really witnessed the consequences of change in the west because the natives have collaborated to maintain the idealistic safety nets into a more private domain. The outcome of post-industrial society may have permitted a person to become more privatized but it has also permitted him to carry his ideals into reality in a more secure way. Through privatization they are safe and free from scrutiny in a way that they never could be by the close knit communities of the past. In a nutshell, the functions of the community, or network, have not fundamentally changed and the consequences of deviating from the norm are just as severe as they were in the past. Indeed, on an idealistic level the ramifications are more severe because they are threatening a more organic network.

Change, then, from idealistic notions has not really occurred, despite the radical social movements over the last three decades. Deviations from the norm, however, still occur and because the 'community' is not as close knit, in a functional sense, but dispersed over a wider area, natives will be all the more reluctant to be involved in caring. They have not grown up to be connected within a small locale. With fewer social bonds (work, kinship and so on) behaviour that conforms to the norm (i.e. is predictable) is all the more important. As Farmer (1979) suggests:

> ... the majority of families express their individuality, outwardly at least, without gross deviations from acceptable behaviour ... conformity to the general norms of society ... and the expression of conformity through participation ... give the family importance as agents of societal cohesion.

Cohesion, again, suggests conformity. Durkheim (1975) argues that society:

> ... is also a power controlling them (individuals).

Hence the ethic of conformity based on societal norms is first enforced within the family. Because the family (or the major themes of its reality) are projected onto the wider society reactions to non-conformity in the society will be rather severe. Those who do not subscribe to cohesiveness threaten society and each group that comprises society. Such threats can occur when a person does not conform to the expectations we have developed about him/her. Many of those expectations are manifest through an unwritten code. For example when a 'neighbour' greets: 'How are you?', the expected response is: 'Fine', 'Very well', 'Mus'n't grumble', and so on. A person is not expected to respond with their life history.

These expectations are rather insidious and envelop role displays. Even though there are no formal classes on manhood every male is expected to act like a man when he reaches a certain age. The norms defined by society present many problems for men. Caring, the theme of this section, does not figure overtly in a man's world. Role models from the media tend to wallow in aggression which creates a kind of inalienable bond between men. The Gibson and Glover characters (in the 'Lethal Weapon' films) are bound together by constantly saving each others lives. It is almost a dyadic form of the 'Pals' battalions developed in the First World War. The Pals battalions relied on a community link between troops prior to grouping them together. Strong stuff this group identity and peer group pressure. Giving a group a single identity is almost like controlling one person. Men seem more prone to this type of group behaviour. Their only chance to share physical contact is through boys' games – men rarely touch each other except through contact sport (Skidmore, 1986). Because men are cultured into such responses (sexuality to the female, aggression to the male) it is hardly surprising that some men can only relate to the world aggressively. This is the tragedy of men, they learn from early socialization that they gain acceptance through aggression, either excellence in sport or knocking the next boy to the ground. Many bullies gain more attention through their bullying activities than they do at other times. Recent news stories reveal the office bully and the office sexual harasser (usually male and both acts of aggression). Attempts to rehabilitate violent offenders tend to try and rechannel the aggression to a more socially acceptable type, such as motorcycle scrambling. The sad aspect of this is that the overtly caring male is stereotyped in society as being effeminate.

The implication here is that there are gender specific qualities and caring is clearly the domain of the female. If a man shows this quality then we have to reclassify him as a wimp or homosexual. An interesting point here is that the most successful film of 1993, signalled as a future cult film, is a work of violence, *Reservoir Dogs*; there are no central female characters and the male leads relate to each other by way of aggression. This then is how men are recognized. There is an identifiable role for each group in society and they are expected to conform to that role or be reclassified. It was suggested above that the world becomes part of us, therefore by protecting the world we are protecting ourself. Hence, reclassifying a person gives meaning to non-conformist behaviour.

CARING

So far we have visited normality. What happens to the person who cannot conform to society's norms? The process of deviance has been touched on in Part One, but this looked at the process rather than the individual. It is relatively easy to offer care to a person who is otherwise like us. But consider the process of change. When a person retires, is made unemployed, becomes ill or is divorced his/her circumstances change. In these cases there are clearly recognized labels that allow others to reclassify the person. However, the person may have to reclassify self, internally, in order to cope with the new existence. Timetables and networks will have been seriously disrupted. Two points of connection with community severed. Being partially disconnected in this way will create a disturbance in everyday behaviour which, in turn, disrupts the lives of other members in the group and 'community'. Using retirement as an exemplar the retired male may attempt to take over some of the role of his spouse, purely to fill his day. She should not mind this because she cares for him. However, rather than helping her he is projecting his 'disconnectedness' onto her and creating a similar state in her.

The assumption is that if a person cares for you they will permit, or should permit, anything. The main focus of care, however, is for self. It is that which facilitates survival, self-care. Next we can care for those who help us feel more secure. One could argue that we only love a person whilst they make us feel good . . . once they stop making us feel good we stop loving them. Hence we are expressing self-love, not love of another person. Therefore, using this argument, a person is the centre of his/her own caring. Just as he projects his world onto others part of his caring will be projected in the process. Thus, those who are part of our social network will receive varying amounts of care based on some kind of return, the contribution they make to our security. Simmel (1950) suggests:

> All contacts among men rest on a schema of giving and returning the equivalence.

Simmel, then would argue that we offer affection and care in the expectation of receiving the same in return. Naturally, in a society which stresses altruistic caring it is difficult to accept that care for self is above all else. Society has developed the notion of a 'superego' or conscience; the desire to follow a code of life because it is right and the denial of taking the abnormal route because it is wrong. Examination of these rules would indicate that they favour the group rather than the individual. If we consider the commandments in context then it is clear that these were designed to make the Jewish tribes more cohesive. Thou shalt not kill a Jew being reduced to Thou shalt not kill over time. Under Hebrew law at the time of the commandments the only persons capable of committing adultery were married women. The married man could have as many concubines as he wanted. Black (1898) argues that the 'love' concept contained in Christianity has been reinforced to strengthen the group effort. The centre of pre-industrial communities was the church with its overt symbolism of loving the fellow man. Black (1898) suggests that by displaying love and friendship for one's fellow man we are expressing our love for God. As early as 1898 Black was suggesting that the decline in caring was due to the change in society and that man prefers to be loved than to give love. He offers a code of friendship that will safeguard society:

> Economics: there should be sharing and giving between friends in all things
> Counselling: friends should give and receive advice willingly
> Help: friends must give help and support in crises
> Moral Control: it is the duty of friendship to moderate behaviour as a form of protection; we should prevent friends from slipping into immoral behaviour
> Pleasure: friends should give each other pleasure by providing a sense of belonging.

Black is attempting to force a structure onto a relationship that defies structure. It has been stressed in Part One that friendship and love are very individual relationships that will have millions of definitions in our society. Black, like many other writers, is analyzing an individual relationship and applying it to the group. This type of analysis, as can be seen from the above, kills the romantic spirit.

Let us return to the theme of the person projecting their world externally; that is, the person projects his/her values onto those others who inhabit his/her community and ascribes them with similar values. Because of the need to preserve that world he/she will identify similar qualities in others. This is done on the basis of 'feeling', not empirical study and, consequently, ideals are safe because they are not subjected to artificial measure. Similarly, caring is an individual emotion. We care for some people and not others, but the 'not-caring' is not malicious or deliberate. Using exchange theory in a more romantic sense we show affection to people we are attracted to, that is those people we feel comfortable with. Because we project our image onto that person and make the assumption that they are like us then we anticipate reciprocal affection. Those we do not care about we do not consciously admit to the private world and expect nothing from them, unless, of course, they try to force entry. In the case of forced entry indifference may turn to active dislike. This concept is crucial to those entering a career in community care. Care is a reciprocal affection. Both partners must want to give and receive care. Like any relationship it cannot flourish if only one party cares, unless the other party is unconscious.

NATURAL CARERS

Every community has a network of caring relationships that evolve naturally. The basic caring unit is that of the family. Parents care for their offspring and the offspring grow to care for their parents in return. The consequences of parental separation and rejection are well documented elsewhere. The implicit duty of family members, as directed by society, is that they care for each other. There is also the bonding that blood relationship creates, particularly between mothers and offspring. There is a folk saying that you can have many fathers but only one mother. Knowledge of natural parents is very important for offspring. Indeed, many adopted children go through considerable effort and angst to trace natural parents. Many children go through private anxiety that they may not really be the offspring of the parents they live with and may eventually be rejected. The point is that this type of basic caring is important for the survival of the individual's psyche; so much so that this aspect of the family is projected to the 'community'. We develop friendships based on similar qualities of caring, but because there are no blood ties these arise from attraction. The scope of networked relationships has been examined previously and will not benefit from further discourse. The main principle of the network is that of mutual care because each member is projecting their own care onto others and believes that he/she is receiving similar care in return. In this context care and affection are blurred. Unlike the functionalist approach it has to be accepted that this is a natural evolution that members accept and do not consciously manufacture. A person's community is composed of a network of natural carers. That caring relationship will be reinforced by several shared links: spending regular time together, using the same amenities, sharing friends and so on.

CARING CAREERS

The caring career suggests something that can be artificially produced. Professionals seem to deny that you have to have some liking for a person before you can care for them. We humans are not that expert at controlling our body language when we dislike a person, regardless of how professional we are. Problems arise because we accept that caring is natural and can be transferred to others automatically. Professionals consequently develop models of care to project onto clients and these will be explored in the next chapter. A caring career, such as that of the parent, is full time. Parents care about their offspring even in their absence. We carry images of our offspring to remind us and when part of our family dies part of each member dies. The professional carer can only ever be part time and/or periodic. The images they carry are case notes rather than photographs and that symbolizes the condition not the person. Caring is person-centred. The people we naturally care for are self-selected; professional carers have people referred to them. Because the choice is eliminated in the professional relationship the process of caring has been mechanized, and this will be examined in the next chapter. Natural caring relationships are not formally timetabled. We do not ascribe one hour per week to be with our friend nor do we only allow mother to telephone at certain times. Natural care flourishes because of its lack of formality, there are no perceived obligations to meet. In the professional caring relationship the problem of transference often occurs; the client is attracted to the therapist. Female clients falling for the male doctor, male clients falling for female doctors, these cases are almost commonplace and the issue of transference will be mentioned in many practice manuals. It need not be some complex mechanism that requires a label. It can arise because we all see caring in a natural context and misread the signs. Members of the opposite sex care for us because they are related or they are attracted. This is the process we have grown to recognize. To reiterate in natural life care and affection are blurred. In the professional world care and attraction become blurred. Consequently guidelines and rules have to be imposed to safeguard both parties and this adds to the artificial nature of the relationship.

The professional caring career then is punctuated by its part time or periodic nature and artificiality. The business of caring on the mechanical level, i.e. when there is a patient who is injured, is relatively easy because we care for the condition. This process in itself has been the subject of much debate and is accused of dehumanizing the medical process. Unfortunately this type of care is focused and not directed to the whole person, it could never be anything else. The dehumanizing debate has been responsible in part for client-centred care. It could be argued that it has deepened the dehumanizing effect. Consider the 'skills' in counselling, specifically 'active listening'. One cannot feign interest, to attempt to do so is insulting to the client. To be interested in a person means that one has to like them. Some counsellors are excellent and have a genuine liking for people. Their success has condemned other practitioners to follow their lead. In this sense caring has been mechanized and misdirected. There is nothing wrong with caring about a condition if that is what a person is good at. Excellent car mechanics care about what they do, they need not care for the driver; builders enjoy constructing houses, they do not have to care for the family who is to live there. Similarly clinicians care about saving life, they do not have to have a genuine interest in the person to do this. We have consistently done the medical model a disservice by attacking it by way of this route.

Human beings, as has been suggested in Part One, are composed of various parts: biology, sociology, psychology and politics. If a person has entered a diabetic coma he/she cannot be counselled out of it, no matter how caring a person is. Similarly a person who feels disconnected from his community cannot be 'treated' in a purely biological sense. Holistic care attempts to place care of the total person on each practitioner. In reality the 'care' of a person should be viewed as a team effort. Real care can only be delivered by real carers. Professional care is hampered by its artificiality and consequently requires those natural carers who excel in offering support on this basis. It is ludicrous to expect all professionals to be able to develop this skill. In an ideal world all professionals would care for their clients, the next chapter will explore why this can never be possible.

This chapter has examined community in terms of an extension of the family. In this context caring has also been reviewed as a quality that occurs naturally and cannot be artificially created. The next chapter will take this theme further and examine the model that professions base their caring approach upon.

REFERENCES

Bell, D. (1956) The theory of mass society. *Commentary*, July.
Bilton, T., Bonnett, T., Jones, P. *et al.* (1987) *Introductory Sociology*, Macmillan, London.
Black, H. (1898) *Friendship*, Hodder and Stoughton, London.
Bramson, L. (1961) *The Political Context of Sociology*, Princeton University Press, New Jersey.
Durkheim, E. (1964) *The Division of Labour in Society*, Free Press, New York.
Durkheim, E. (1975) *Suicide*, Routledge and Kegan Paul, London.
Farmer, M. (1979) *The Family*, Longman, London.
Frankenberg, R. (1975) *Communities in Britain*, Penguin, Harmondsworth, Middlesex.
Goode, W.J. (1964) *The Family*, Prentice Hall, New Jersey.
Laing, R.D. (1971) *Self and Others*, Penguin, Harmondsworth, Middlesex.
Lorenz, K. (1967) *On Aggression*, Methuen, London.
Parker, S. (1976) *The Sociology of Leisure*, Allen and Unwin, London.
Rope, J.A. (1969) Friendship and highrise living. University of Birmingham, unpublished research report.
Simmel, G. (1950) *The Sociology of Georg Simmel*, Free Press, New York.
Skidmore, D. (1986) The sociology of friendship. University of Keele, PhD Thesis.
Tonnies, F. (1955) *Community and Association*, Routledge and Kegan Paul, London.
Weber, M. (1949) *The Methodology of the Social Sciences*, Free Press, New York.
Wilmot, P. (1963) *The Evolution of Community*, Routledge and Kegan Paul, London.

CHAPTER 8

Mothers and fathers

The first caring relationship that most people experience is that of the parent-child relationship. Nietzsche (1977) suggests that all relationships are master-slave relationships. What Nietzsche means here is that each partner will slip into a master role and then a slave role depending on the circumstances. Some relationships, like the parent-child relationship, are characterized by one party being the predominant master. Children gain power in other ways, such as feigning illness. It has already been suggested, in Chapter 7, that the family has clear role expectations of its members. Parents are dominant:

male breadwinner = provider and lawgiver
female complementary = support and carer
child = to receive care and obey rules.

This model facilitates caring since everyone knows their place. It also becomes the model of caring that we project into our world.

The second model of caring arises out of friendship. This relationship is, as has been discussed, an extension of self-care. In general we ascribe our personal qualities to our friends, hence caring for them is not difficult since it is like caring for self.

The third model of caring arises out of sexual love. Blau (1967) argues that this type of relationship develops through an imbalance of exchange into mutual attraction. The parties of this relationship gain pleasure by spending time together. However, spending time together becomes crucial to the relationship because if either deliberately absent themselves from the other it advertises non-attraction. The activities within this type of relationship are more 'person-centred' in a physical sense than the previous models we have constructed.

There is, of course, a blurring between these models of care. In some cases the sexual model is extended to the family with devastating results. That which we normally accept is guided by unwritten rules as well as formal laws. Consequently there are ideal types of caring which provide a framework for social encounters. The most significant ideal type is the parent-child model which is natural and expected to withstand any crises. It could be argued that this is the model adopted by professional carers. Consider first of all the traditional view of the medical model. The doctor is the father, the nurse the mother and the patient the child.

The implication is that this is a caring relationship with the doctor providing and giving the laws; the nurse supports him in this and is the prime giver of care, the patient obeys and receives care. In return he is expected to be grateful.

The traditional view of the father was one of a somewhat transient figure in the life of a child. Most of their waking hours he would spend at work and offer fleeting visits now and again. He could, in this respect, be used as a threat to unruly children, as in 'Wait 'til your father gets home!' The hospital doctor, particularly the consultant, can be seen to mirror this role. They are transient, but significant, figures in the patient's career. It is they who make the rules and can gainsay a discharge date. The unruly patient can be threatened with: 'If you don't take the tablets I'll just have to let the doctor know.' Unlike most families, however, this father can delegate his authority to surrogate fathers, such as registrars and housemen. The patient, then, has to please several fathers by his progress.

The traditional view of the mother is one of the female who devotes her time to the total care of her children and is respectful and supportive of her husband. The traditional view of the nurse is one of the female, the handmaiden to the doctor. It is an image that is difficult to shatter. From the patient's point of view the nurse is present around the clock to care for him should this be necessary. He will witness her respect for the doctor when he carries out his rounds and, just like parents, they will have their private moments from which children are excluded. The nurse is the person who has the ear of the lawgiver but will conspire with her charges to the benefit of them. Similarly the mother is the go-between in the father-child relationship and she will collude with her children out of father's earshot.

The traditional view of the child is one of a dutiful and respectful offspring who obeys his parents and strives to make them proud of him. He is passive in the everyday decision making of family life. Disrespect or deviation from that which is expected of him will result in a momentary withdrawal of care and affection. Similarly the patient is expected to be passive in the everyday decision-making process that goes on about his care. He is expected to follow instructions, receive care and make his medical parents proud by striving to get well. Any deviation from the norm will result in a momentary withdrawal of care and affection (Stockwell, 1972). The patient relationship with the doctor mirrors that of the father-child in its formality. Children tend to be far more informal with mothers and will develop a banter with them, sharing jokes and developing inclusive behaviour. This is quite rare with fathers (remember we are concerned with traditional and ideal type families here). Similarly patients will often develop a more informal relationship with the nurses on the ward. There is often a blurring of the mother-lover image for male patients here which will lead to the child teasing the mother. In this context the legend of Oedipus lives. The nurse has become firmly established as a figure of sexual fantasy. The type of banter arising from this relationship would never be established with the doctor. However, the female patient may blur the father-lover image.

These are the natural models that professionals and patients carry with them to the encounter. Added to this are a collection of formal and informal rules that have developed over years. The formal rules are based on the ethical concerns for care delivery and the informal rules are developed through experience. On the formal side there are rules governing the sexual behaviour of professionals involved in care delivery and any sexual encounter with a patient can lead to the professional losing the right to practice. This aspect of the code of practice immediately demands that practitioners do not see their clients as people, for they have to deny their sexuality. In order to protect themselves many doctors and nurses do, indeed, see conditions rather than people. The protection of the sexual integrity of the patient is, of course, very important. The patient is usually in crisis and very susceptible to outside influence (Caplan, 1964). Hence, the practitioner could abuse their position here. The conundrum is that by law practitioners are encouraged not to see patients as people (or adults) whilst at the same time being expected to take a patient-centred approach. It is hinted, here, that one way of coping is to view patients as children. Children are similarly protected by law concerning any sexual approaches made against them by parents.

Here, then, are two points of reference that place an imbalance within the professional-client relationship: the model of care that each brings to the encounter with them and the need to safeguard the sexuality of the patient. Both points of reference facilitate the image of patient as child. Children are not expected to be consulted about their rearing. They have, after all, no experience of life and consequently need much direction. If patients are seen in the same way, and we must not think that all this occurs on a conscious level, then it would be quite incongruent to involve them in decisions about their treatment. To develop this further, the deeper a patient is in that state of normlessness the more childlike he becomes. Skidmore (1979, 1980) differentiates between the levels of medical care (Chapter 4) and describes how the patient in the medical nucleus is almost totally passive. Attempts to involve him in the treatment process are rarely successful. The patient, then, will bring a variable amount of childlikeness with him depending on the encounter. Visiting the GP will cause the client to become more mature as he grows through the process. GPs come to be viewed as informed family friends (Skidmore, 1979). The community nurse, however, is an agent of the hospital and, as such, is invested with more parental powers.

The childlikeness is not static, of course. Just as the relationship with one's GP develops, a patient with a chronic illness will come to know a great deal about it and be less childlike in some encounters.

MESSIANIC PARENTS

The parental image of the professional can, however, be reinforced by the messianic syndrome. In short this is developed in professionals by the elation they receive through the power of the healing process. It is akin to the enigmatic laying-on of hands carried out by the Messiah or the 'who was that masked therapist?' image. The messianic impulse causes the professional to gather a mantle of mystery around him. Illich (1976) calls this a priest like quality. It also means keeping one's knowledge secret from the child so that the child is always in awe of the parents' ability to care, and of course extremely grateful. The formal process of care delivery has facilitated the messianic aspect of care. Like any other group doctors and their colleagues develop a style of language that becomes inclusive. They may address a patient in this language, because it has become so commonplace that it is thought all the natives understand. This bewilders the patient. Our society associates elaborated speech with intelligence and expressed intelligence is quite frightening since it invites a person to play a game of which the rules are unknown. Simplistically it is the process of investing trust and respect in a person because they can use and understand very long words. In the early days of medical training this 'skill' was actively encouraged because it was thought that it would convince patients that serious scientific thought was going on.

The need to formalize care has been necessary in order to train people to deliver care. But this is not the care we encounter in 'caring' relationships and it does need to be separated. The professional can only relate to practitioner status through a process of categorization. The diagnosis is helpful in offering a framework for planning treatment. The condition is, quite rightly, at the centre of the diagnostic process and based on the majority of presenting symptoms. This process has worked for the common good for many years. Problems have arisen with this process when an individual focus has been enforced upon it. Individual care is a noble principle but not very practical. Economy of 'care' delivery demands a standard process. Attempts to enforce the tenets of natural care onto the process devalue both. Caring is essentially 'felt' about another person. To some extent it is a reflection of how we feel about ourselves because we can make predictions about the person we care about.

On the mechanistic level this is exactly what the diagnosis achieves for the practitioner. It allows him to make predictions about the patient and, consequently, facilitates mechanistic caring. Since the predictions only concern the condition a person has, then that is where caring will be directed. This should not be problematical since, at this level of care, we are concerned with repairing so that the person can resume normal functions. Mechanistic caring favours acute intervention. Acute intervention can never rise above mechanistic levels since there can never be exchange within a long-term relationship. It concerns itself with normal people who have a problem that needs solving but will return to being normal people. Investment in anything other than this would be fruitless. On the basic level we are not structured to offer the same level of affection to everyone we meet. Indeed, just as in the professional relationship, our affections are governed by certain rules. We are expected to have just one sexual partner at any one time, to honour parents above all others and have a few special friends. Society, then, suggests a finite quantity to the amount of affection, and with it caring, we can offer. This has become part of our world, the world we project onto others. Since professionals are human beings they are bound by the same rules. Hence, to expect that they invest real care onto those they visit is a nonsense.

Treatment programmes for the chronically ill are a different matter. This is the very area where caring for the person could be fostered. Unfortunately the chronically ill present other problems. In crude terms they have ceased to be normal. The ideal type of sick role suggests that a person will get better. The notion of chronicity implies a change of identity and something about which we can no longer make predictions. The desire to care, then, is offset by the inability to predict. The normal progression of 'illness' experienced by the patient/client has also been disrupted, he no longer knows what to expect and will, initially, seek security in childlikeness. The mechanistic health care system will, however, seek to give him increasing responsibility for his condition once he is confirmed as chronic. The acute focus of care delivery is not geared to handing over responsibility. Thus, the first feeling the patient may have could be analogous to the rejected child. He may become petulant and not comply with medication in order to receive attention from the parents. We do learn from an early age that being ill offers political gains. We can gain more attention from our parents by being ill, we can escape punishment for mischievousness when we are ill. Certainly being ill forces communication between self and those who profess to care.

So far it has been suggested that all parties approach the health care arena with the parent-child model. Because of the 'part time' nature of health care delivery this is rarely successful as a relationship. It is further complicated when care moves into the 'community' since the client is expected to have the dual roles of part time patient (child) and adult at most other times. In addition the practitioner is invading the client's home, where the client has authority. When the client was a patient in hospital he was on foreign territory and needed the guidance to escape that country. Now he is expected to be a visitor in his own country. This is stimulated by the imagery that the practitioner brings with her (female for clarity) into the encounter; she is an agent of that other country where he (the client, male for clarity) was once lost. She may have the power to take him back to that other country if he breaks the rules, just like parents can send you to your room. To reinforce this aspect a whole collection of foster parents and step-parents will feel the need to get involved in some way.

FOSTER PARENTS

In this context foster parents are those people who naturally care about the sick person and feel that they should do something. Friends, relatives and neighbours will offer help, at least in the short term, because that is the nature of that person's relationship with them. It is, of course, anticipated that the person would do the same for them. This rallying round of the lay network will confirm the sickness location of a person. Like other foster parents this involvement in care is seen to be a short term measure until the person is self-sufficient or the natural parents return. The implication here is that care by a community will not go on indefinitely whereas care in the community may. There is, then, a natural life span for foster parents and if caring is invested totally in this relationship the long term sick could easily become orphans. Certainly the natural parents (doctors and nurses) are much more distanced. The doctor may now be analogous with the father who works on the oil-rig, only visiting periodically (outpatients clinic) and the nurse with the mother who has had her children taken into care and is allowed to visit once per week. The community network will gradually detach from caring when the illness is protracted. Blood relatives will continue much longer. There are documented cases of daughters giving up their lives to look after a sick mother or father. The more common model today is to have the parent placed in a residential home.

The natural or professional parents, of course, have all the authority and may even use foster parents as conspirators. Skidmore and Friend (1984) discovered evidence of relatives conspiring with the community nurse. There could be, then, a slight change in role here and the foster parent becomes the go-between from client to professional parent. The foster parent will also be used to police the instructions delivered: 'Make sure he takes his medication'. Such responsibility will give the foster parent a degree of power over the client and may distance the relationship somewhat. The foster parent is acting out of concern but it draws the relationship into an arena that is no longer predictable. The client is being forced into a childlike role and expected to comply with the rules of others whilst in his own home. This home is where he projects his private world and realizes his ideals. Such actions may cause him to question his construction of reality, thereby adding to the problem. In short informal carers should not be abused by investing them with a policing function. A further problem is that by using informal carers in this way it formalizes the relationship. It removes the motive of wanting to spend time together and reduces it to one of having a duty to carry out. This stimulates the doubt in the client that his friend is forced to spend time with him and he has become a burden in his own community. Let us not forget that we have all collected evidence regarding how our community feels about those who make excessive demands on others.

The move to give a person care in the community sends contradictory messages to that person. Either the person is not ill enough to merit total care or he/she is beyond professional help. The lay community has a store of case histories of natives being sent home to die. For the person disabled by a stroke the message is clearly that 'we have done all we can'. The newly disabled person is permanently discharged to the care of foster parents. The consequences of this new identity have been discussed in Chapter 5. The newly disabled become emigres in their own countries because of their new identities, the changes in their social networks and the loss of independence. For this person, whose disability is permanent but who may have been given the hope of improvement, even the daytrippers eventually stop visiting. Their care may be devolved to step-parents, which, in some cases, may become a process of secondary normalization.

STEP-PARENTS

Step-parents are, on the one hand, those groups who form associations because they either suffer from the condition or are relatives of sufferers. On the other hand they represent the increasing number of alternative therapists (aromatherapists, reflexologists and so on). Whilst, in many ways, a tribute to the humanistic side of people they are, at the same time, an indictment that the health service has either deserted them or failed to provide an effective service. On the economic level step-parents are an excellent alternative to formal services because they negate the need to provide services in the future. Alternative therapists are gaining increasing trade from those persons who are placed on waiting lists as well as those who have been rejected by the health services. Consider the 'self-help' groups, those groups united by experience of a disease or dysfunction. Such groups can develop into highly structured organizations and lobby for better conditions for those they represent. MIND is an obvious example. The tragedy is that these groups have to form in the first place in a so-called caring society. Practitioners should be at the forefront of advocacy for sufferers. We find ourselves back on the doorstep of acute care. In a service that is geared towards short term care, it is inevitable that such groups arise. Even when the formal carers are involved in community care it is only part time care. The step-parent offers legitimacy to the sufferer's condition. They are either receiving support from an organization or receiving therapy from an alternative practitioner. Both activities advertise a willingness to try and return to a normal state. There is an antithesis regarding self-help groups and that is that it may work against the urge to return to a 'normal' state by claiming that there is nothing wrong with having the condition. This can lead to support for the normalization debate which, in reality, is nothing more than a form of neglect. The principles of normalization have been liberally examined in Part One.

The position of step-parents as an alternative to formal care is supported by the message given by a discharge into the community. Acute medicine carries the message that when you are discharged you are well on the way to getting well. Consider the person with a broken leg, discharge into the community means that he/she is getting close to the day when the 'cast' comes off. The person with the broken leg also carries the symbol of acute care with them. We can witness the white cast on his/her leg and consequently make allowances for that person, reassured that he/she will soon be 'well' again. Indeed, the symbol can be a focus of conversation and give access to new relationships. Conversely, a person with a visible chronic condition is unlikely to attract conversation about his/her condition whilst he/she is present. The main reaction attracted is avoidance and the health care system has not provided the skills to deal with that. When there is no visible deformity suspicion is attracted: 'Is he/she really ill?'

Diabetic neuropathy can be very debilitating. The sufferer will experience pains in the legs and lack of energy for anything up to 2 years from the onset. There will be days when the sufferer feels alright and may engage in everyday activities, only to be 'laid-up' again the next day. Bouts of depression often accompany the condition which can suggest a totally psychological problem to the lay-carers. Similarly the sporadic periods of 'normality' suggest that the person is really okay and the condition is a sham. For the sufferer there is a sense that they will never get well again. The diabetes cannot be cured, that is certain, and it is that condition which has caused the present state. The main symptom is the pain and aching in the limbs and that is not visible to an outsider. Anyone can claim to have a pain and if they have to take a pill, we know from the media that they work. However, sufferers often use their pain to seek reassurance. That is not to say that they do not feel pain, they certainly do. However, the focus of conversation regarding the pain is a way of seeking explanation and reassurance about the condition. Unfortunately when people keep talking about their condition we grow suspicious about its very existence; professionals and layfolk alike. The treatment of pain by the professional is quite strange. Although it is recognized as existing it is treated in a uniform way and the psychological aspects are almost ignored. Janis (1971) explored the postoperative use of analgesia and found that it could be controlled by giving total information prior to the operation. Basically patients arrive for an operation with the belief that they are going to be very well after it. Invasive surgery always creates pain and when the patient recovered from the anaesthetic and awoke into a world of pain, they were convinced something had gone wrong. When they reported the pain, they were given treatment but no reassuring explanations. Janis (1971) discovered that preparing the patient with accurate information led to a reduction in the amount of analgesia and an earlier discharge. Another aspect that tends to be ignored is that people have different pain thresholds and experience more or less discomfort. People also experience psychological pain in similar ways. Psychological pain can be caused by any intervention but particularly when the intervention is terminated but the condition continues.

SINGLE PARENTS

There is a class of person discharged into the community who will not receive the attention of either foster parents or step-parents. These are the people who have to parent themselves because they have become disconnected from society. These people are not confined to the chronically mentally ill category and have representatives from all the chronic conditions. They are the social refugees and have become lost in the system. For this group care in the community is very part time. They may receive a 5-minute visit in the hostel every 2 weeks to be given an injection or receive a supportive visit for half an hour every week. This type of activity may advertise an interest by the professional but does it count as caring? Indeed, the visits may even prevent them developing social networks with other residents of the hostel because it advertises that there is something wrong with them. The plight of this group has been explored in some depth in Part One. Briefly it is from this group that the problem cases will arise that the Minister of Health intends to appoint psychiatric probation officers for. In August 1993 the Minister announced that there would be no increase in community nurses to allow for the additional duties. Consequently one must conclude that services will be directed from other needy groups in order to take of this duty. This is merely the transfer of neglect and no doubt in several years' time another problem group will arise. The single parents have been manufactured through our neglect as a caring society. The policies currently being instituted by the government compound that neglect by removing their status as people.

CARE IN THE COMMUNITY

Care in the community involves practitioners intruding into the client's world. Given that they have usually received training within an institution they will carry part of their world with them (Golan, 1978). District nurses, for example, still wear uniforms, the case is also indicative of the professional status. Craddock (1962) suggests that clients feel more comfortable about taking their problems to a professional who is community based; he refers to the GP. Skidmore and Friend (1984) discovered similar evidence with self-referrals to community psychiatric services that were primary health care based. Only 5% of new referrals to hospital-based community psychiatric services were self-referrals, whereas 25% of new referrals in the primary health care base were self-referred. In Part One it was argued that people still feel that they have some control about services offered at local level. Consequently, from a political point of view, the base for care in the community should be local. The principles of locality management appear to be moving in the right direction here. Care in the community implies that the client should take an active part in the treatment. In order to facilitate this, the politics of the exchange (from passivity to activity) have to be well managed. Having the service on one's doorsteps, as has been the case with the GP, is a step in the right direction.

Unfortunately many of the self-referees to psychiatric community services have been labelled 'the worried well'. These are the cases whose psychological dysfunction is stimulated by sociological causes, such as divorce. The publicity surrounding the 'neglected' long term mentally ill has led to services been directed away from this group. Subsequently they have received chemotherapy from the GP which has led to a host of psychiatric iatrogenesis: making demands on the GP's time for counselling and becoming dependent on the drugs. The GP's time is precious and he/she has a crucial role as a generic practitioner who can refer persons to the specialist area where they will receive the right attention. The group of people making demands because of a lack of service interfere with that role. It does not make economic sense to redirect resources in this way because the key players will have their function hampered. With the institution of psychiatric probation officers this group will undoubtedly increase. The major problem with this is that it reduces the amount of care in the community by turning the health centre into a mini-institution. By this one means that a certain group of persons will become dependent on the health centre for an increasing amount of problems at an increasing amount of time. Skidmore (1979) reported that GPs found that this group of people eventually started to consult the GP about every aspect of life from taking out a mortgage to problems with children at school. This is the type of dependence fostered by institutions. With regard to acute care it is acceptable. For example, a person with appendicitis has to receive total care and have his affairs managed on his behalf until he is well. Institutionalization is not likely to occur in such a case because the person is inoculated by the knowledge that:

1. he has a known condition for which there is a recognized service and treatment;
2. he is receiving intervention to relieve the condition;
3. he will be discharged from formal care when well.

In addition the professionals are working with the same knowledge and will have a definite timetable of care. The person in the 'worried well' group has no such inoculation. He/she feels unwell but can gain access to no recognized service, can gain no idea about total discharge which advertises when one will be well. However, at the same time he/she must be ill because of the continued prescriptions. The condition, being secondary, has arisen from crisis during which a person is unable to make decisions. The person has been assisted here by the friendly neighbourhood GP. It is a case of 'for the want of a nail . . .'. The fairly acute condition has been turned into a chronic condition for the lack of an effective community service. The ramifications are twofold: a person's life is damaged and the GP service is becoming clogged-up. Professionals have been misled by the belief that institutionalization was created by institutions and the answer is to transfer people into community settings. Institutionalization is the consequence of 'dispowering' people when they should be empowered.

Consequently disempowerment can happen in any setting. Mere discharge into the community will not eradicate the condition. Care in the community has to employ empowerment in its treatment regimens, whatever condition is being treated. It is only through empowerment that a person can make decisions about his or her own life. Hence, on the political level care in the community should be a partnership where seniority is gradually handed over to the client through empowerment. This has to be realistic, of course, and some clients can never be empowered. On the purist level care in the community can only be offered to those capable of independent living. Those who require specialist registers and monitoring of that order are arguably unfit for the community. Purist argument is a dangerous line to take because it reinforces the classification debate. If we can be black and white about who should receive care in the community we can similarly be clear on who should not. The problem lies in the professionals' inability to deal with the person. Conditions are impersonal and much easier to make decisions about. Care in the community is not about conditions but people. People react in different ways to the same condition. However when a handful of people suffering from a condition commit serious social acts it is the condition that receives bad press, hence everyone with that condition is classified as dangerous. The worst excesses of this process were witnessed in the mental hospitals with the secure wards. Patients were often sent there for punishment and would mirror the behaviour expected of them. In essence, then, care in the community must refer to the person and not specific conditions. This presents the problem that most practitioners are taught to relate to conditions and not people and, unfortunately, this is the most effective way of dealing with large numbers. This makes the need for client empowerment all the more essential.

ACUTE AND CHRONIC CARE

It is becoming apparent in this debate that care in the community attempts to cover two areas, the acute and the chronic. The present system is partially suitable for acute work since there is a clear timetable of involvement. In many cases it is highly successful and perhaps that success has led to the same principle being applied to the chronic arena. The inoculation factor of many acute cases will ensure empowerment and will not lead to professional resistance of same. There is a natural end to the carer's career in acute community work. Different approaches are required for chronic work, however. For the reasons offered in this text a person with a chronic condition becomes 'dispowered' and, hence, passive in all things. The dispowered client becomes a willing victim of institutionalization which will not require professionals to create and maintain it. When a person becomes passive it encourages others to take over their lives, the step-parents and foster parents. These people will take on the day-to-day decisions about how that person lives his/her life. Over time the person will learn to be helpless within his/her own home. Because of the part time nature of care in the community it is not suitable for a major part of chronic conditions and the concept of care by the community should be explored. Chronic conditions will require treatment for a protracted period and often for life. For this reason maxim empowerment is essential where possible. The classic example is the insulin-dependent diabetic who is given full responsibility for his/her treatment, even unto modifying insulin dosage. That empowerment has been possible because there is a highly structured diabetic service in the formal arena. The diabetic services in many areas of the country could be highlighted as models of practice for care in and by the community. The objective is that the client takes over full responsibility for care and the family is educated into a supporting role rather than a caring role. There is no doubt that diabetes is a chronic condition and yet the person-centred style of intervention allows sufferers to be totally integrated into their communities. That style is punctuated by empowerment rather than having professionals visit to do things to the person. The professional is a source of reference. In other conditions the involvement of professionals can distance the person from his/her condition. It is something a person only has when the nurse visits and is only important at that time. The process of empowerment is the process of giving the client responsibility for his/her condition. Diabetes is a lifestyle issue concerning diet and activity, it could not be treated on a part time basis. Perhaps if the same philosophy were to be adopted by those treating people with a long term psychosis social integration may occur.

The person with a psychosis, albeit under control, is never really trusted to dispense his/her medication. They could be taught to give their own injections which is possible for deep intramuscular injections. If they cannot be trusted, arguably they are not ready for care in the community. Each case has to be assessed on the personal level and cannot be judged by the expectation of the condition. One line of argument is that 'psychotics' cannot be trusted to give their own medication. Surely that is their responsibility just as much as the diabetic. The consequences of not giving one's own insulin are far more drastic and dire than not giving a long acting phenothiazine. The fact that this group are given their injections by others advertises that they are not capable of doing so. It is, of course, too simplistic to think that responsibility can be transferred to all persons who have psychoses, some will be totally incapable. Similarly it is just as simplistic to believe that responsibility can not be transferred to any of them. This principle extends to all chronic conditions.

CARE BY THE COMMUNITY

Care by the community does not necessarily mean enlisting informal carers to carry out the role of the professional. In essence, care by the community is the transference of the responsibility of care into the client's world. That may mean using the client's network or self-care by the client. Remember communities are personally defined. It does involve empowerment and almost total withdrawal by the professional. The transference of 'caring' may be to the client and/or significant others. Whichever process is involved it is not a cheap alternative if it is to be successful. When others are involved, step or foster parents, they will require some education if secondary conditions are to be avoided. The messianic syndrome can be stimulated in informal carers as well as professionals. The need to be needed is a powerful influence. Power over others is in itself a corruptive influence. As Lewis (1971) asks:

> Have we discovered some new reason why, this time, power should not corrupt as it has done before?

Therefore, care by the community will involve a major programme of education and training. We can assume that some people care for others, we cannot assume that all people care for all. The professional has a significant role in caring by the community in that he/she has to direct the programme of care whilst, at the same time, safeguarding the identity of the client.

The professional community carer has a major problem when getting involved with care by the community. He/she is immediately confronted with the problem of who expects care from whom. Given the idealistic basis of friendships (explored in Part One) can we realistically expect friends to offer care. Similarly, given the individualistic nature of humanity some persons may expect more care than others; indeed, some may demand no care by others. Care by the community is a totally personal construct. A person may feel that his/her very world is threatened by allowing members of his/her community to become involved in caring.

Caring by the community, then, will involve some kind of functional assessment by the professional. This will give the professional a perception of the client's community. For example one cannot assume that the condition affects only one person. In order to develop a programme to facilitate care by the community the practitioner needs to know:

1. How many significant persons are involved in this community?
   This knowledge has implications regarding who should be involved in planning and information exchange.
2. What are the presenting problems?
   This concerns the major dysfunction that impacts on the life of the person and those around him/her.
3. Are there any related problems dependent upon the outcome of the presenting problem?
   For example are the person's relationships likely to break down if the problem is not resolved?
4. Who defined the problem and was responsible for the client seeking help?
   An important issue because it reveals whether or not the client is empowered regarding dealing with the condition. If the relatives or other members of a network have instigated referral it could imply learned helplessness or scapegoating.
5. What are the consequences of non intervention?
   Basically do you need to be involved as a professional? This is a personal question for the professional since they cannot deal with all problems. Should the therapist refer to another agency?
6. What are the losses and gains if the problem is resolved?
   Remember the therapist is trying to preserve the client's social network. Consider the problem of institutionalization in the chronically mentally ill. The resolution was felt to be integration into the community but the loss is a total integration of the social network

and potential social isolation. This issue can only be explored at a personal level.

7. Is the problem situation located?
    In other words does the problem get worse in certain situations or is there no apparent reasons for the occurrence.

8. Self-fulfilment.
    How comfortable is the person with their community? Do they feel in control or controlled?

9. Influence of significant others.
    How intense are the person's social networks? The therapist will require a knowledge of the person's community in order to gauge who should be involved in care by the community.

10. Evidence of denial.
    Is the client and/or his/her community refusing to accept that there is a problem?

11. Strength of the social network.
    This knowledge will inform whether or not self-care in totality or with the support of others is required. One cannot assume that every person has a social network or that they wish to be involved in caring. The diabetic model is an example here, where they actively canvas the views of those significant others.

12. If there is a social network, are there mutual strengths?
    This is where the genuine aspect of caring can be realized. If members of the social network enjoy carrying out activities with the client these could be utilized in the care programme.

13. Social aspects.
    This is concerned with the location of the client in a social network. For example is he/she an influence to or influenced by others. Will the network reinforce progress or hamper it? Is the problem secondary to a dysfunctional social life?

14. Treatment/resolution.
    Does another agency need to be involved? Is there an agreed and identified problem? Does it suit the network for the client to remain in the present condition? Can the problem be resolved in the community? In other words is it a question of acute or chronic care? That is, treatment in or by the community. Should the client be facilitated in his/her acceptance of the problem?
    (freely adapted from Butterworth and Skidmore, 1983)

It is argued that this type of analysis, on an ongoing basis, will help the practitioner to be more person-centred. Given that a person is the centre of his/her own community then a person is central to care in and by the community. Using this functional approach should eradicate the need to use labels which are incongruent with the person-centred approach. Functional assessment involves observed performance of deficits or advantages that people have (Butterworth and Skidmore, 1983). Naturally this will involve more than the therapist in assessment and can be a time-consuming task. However, such assessment is essential if the process of community care is to be successful.

Following assessment the professional is required to help the client, and any significant others, devise a treatment programme. Note that the professional helps to devise the programme since the process of empowerment should start from day one. Central to any programme is being totally honest with the 'community' – the client and significant members of the social network – honest with regard to what can realistically be achieved. If improvement is unlikely this should be declared because it will take the intervention programme in a different direction to that when improvement is a possibility. Similarly the programme has to be person specific. There is no point in utilizing a programme that requires an active client if the client is naturally passive. Finally the responsibility for care by the community must be handed over to the community.

Central to this discourse is the notion that 'communities' are highly personalized. They exist in as much as a person wills them to exist, as part of that person's construction of reality. The professional cannot make the assumption that it does exist. Being individual some persons may decide that it does not exist. Skidmore (1986) found this to be the case with friendship, albeit in a minority of subjects. The same could be true of community and this will have implications for how the person is treated. This cannot be revealed without entering into dialogue with a client. If he/she reports social isolation then that is his/her community. The idealistic image of community cannot be created artificially for therapeutic reasons. Some people prefer their own company. Naturally this will present as a major problem if the condition is one of major disability and care in or by the community requires the assistance of a foster parent. In such cases residential care may be the only answer. Professionals must not fall into the trap of believing that community care is the successful outcome and anything else is a failure. That which is best for the client and its achievement is the success. Enforcing any regimen which spoils a person's quality of life is the failure.

Another important feature of care by the community is that of caring for the carers. One must not lose sight of the fact that those people who act as foster parents or step-parents, even though voluntary, will have additional stress introduced into their lives. They had a life before they became a carer and still have to get on with it. The professional can at least switch off when off duty, the informal carer may never feel off duty. That is not to say that the professional is not stressed by their role, the literature on burnout is testimony to their stress. There is a difference, however, in that the professional has knowledge to support any intervention he/she is involved in. The informal carer will only have second hand knowledge and additional duties to perform. There will also be changes in role to cope with, the son looking after the mother for example. Support of the informal carer involves far more than mere education. Often it will involve a counselling service.

Community care is only a cheap option when it is a facade for neglect, it cannot be carried out on the cheap. Decanting any group into society with the assumption that someone somewhere will pick up the caring is both unethical and immoral. The amount of services demanded in the community has steadily increased without an equivalent rise in personnel. The numbers of health visitors, district nurses, community psychiatric nurses and community nurses for persons with learning difficulties has declined in real terms. Putting health services on a trust basis has led to health care being managed in monetary terms. That places caring on a footing where the person is less important than the cost. It is rather like the banks who profess that people matter, until you reach your credit limit. Similarly, a health service trust can put people first until the money gets tight. In a truly caring society there is no price to be put on a quality of life. In reality we have to reassess our meaning of caring.

The definition of care is 'to feel concern or interest, to have a regard or liking for . . .' (Oxford English Dictionary, 1985). There is, however, an alternative meaning: 'mental suffering, burdened state of mind arising from fear, doubt or concern . . .' (Oxford English Dictionary, 1985). Without an investment in resources it is possible that the latter definition will be paramount. In short we are in danger of spreading mental suffering throughout society with the care in the community policies.

This chapter has examined the implications of care in and by the community, the next chapter will attempt to draw all the themes together. In this way it is hoped that an ideological framework for community care will evolve. It is perhaps worthy of mentioning again that this is not a guide to practice. The issues raised herein are speculations intended to stimulate debate. The only issue that the author would fiercely protect is that the person is central to community care, not policies or blanket practice strategies. The following chapter will explore the notion that we may be a kingdom of orphans.

REFERENCES

Blau, P.M. (1967) *Exchange and Power in Social Life*, Wiley, London.
Butterworth, C.A. and Skidmore, D. (1983) *Caring for the Mentally Ill in the Community*, Croom Helm, London.
Caplan, G. (1964) *Principles of Preventative Psychiatry*, Tavistock, London.
Craddock, D. (1962) *A Family Doctor's Day*, H.K. Lewis, London.
Golan, N. (1978) *Treatment in Crisis Situations*, Macmillan, London.
Illich, I. (1976) *Limits to Medicine*, Penguin, Harmondsworth, Middlesex.

Janis, I. (1971) *Stress and Frustration*, Harcourt Brace, New York.

Lewis, C.S. (1971) *Undeceptions*, Bles, London.

Nietzsche, F. (1977) *A Nietzsche Reader*, Penguin, Harmondsworth, Middlesex.

Skidmore, D. (1979) Anxiety in medical arenas, Cranfield Institute of Technology, MSc Dissertation.

Skidmore, D. (1980) *The Hidden Machine*, Verus, Bournmouth.

Skidmore, D. (1986) The sociology of friendship. University of Keele, PhD Thesis.

Skidmore, D. and Friend, W. (1984) CPNs and base location. The Manchester Metropolitan University, research report.

Stockwell, F. (1972) *The Unpopular Patient, RCN Research Project*, Vol. 1, no. 2, RCN, London.

CHAPTER 9

A kingdom of orphans?

Chapter 1, The geography of being argued that when a person felt located within a particular 'network' then that was his/her community. From this location he/she developed a sense of identity and belonging. Furthermore a person was able to develop a feeling of predictability about his/her life and those persons who shared it. In turn this offered security since a person felt connected and had an identity that was 'recognized' by the 'community'. This was labelled 'personhood'. It is argued that this sense of location is crucial if a person is to successfully relate to society. The Conservative Impulse (Marris, 1974) provides a framework whereby a person can meet most encounters and function effectively.

The location of a person, it is suggested, is the culminative effect of his/her biology, sociology, psychology and politics and these elements are constantly modified by the person's journey through life when future actions are influenced by the past and present. The process of social learning provides a person with a collection of roles that provide a framework to enable the person to structure various encounters. A role provides a code of behaviour and a degree of predictability to any encounter where the role is appropriate. It is suggested that this is Nietzsche's (1977) notion of forcing order onto natural chaos. This argument was developed to suggest that a person had both a private and a public self. The private self contained the individual and the public, the person. Schutz (1962) argues that we are born individuals but become persons through the process of socialization; a person being a socially desirable type. The private self is the cause of a person believing that they are the centre of their own world, but the mechanisms present in society enforce a person to 'act' a series of roles that normally prevents the individual influencing society.

A further mechanism society uses to reinforce group behaviour is the timetable. That is, a structure that suggests a natural and uniform progression over time, e.g. from childhood to adulthood. The timetable demands conformity to those behaviours expected. The timetable suggests that the future is an extension of the past, since role sets are devised through history and tradition.

These themes were carried forward into Chapter 2 and it was argued that they were projected onto a wider society. Aspects of the ideals that a person uses to construct his/her reality are identified as being congruent with others in a person's atlas of existence and these come to be seen as evidence of 'normality'. Certain benchmarks of normality are laid down by society as a marker for standard behaviour. Marriage and family are seen to be constants that preserve society. The structure of society also introduces a system of inequality in most societies and this, in turn, produces a notion of the 'normal' society which is fair and just. The argument was presented that this is, in fact, the falsehood of society and that the reality was a series of overstrung tightropes that we are normally, and willingly, blind to. This is often manifest by the concept of 'knowing'. When we claim to know a person or situation we are projecting our private self into the public arena. This is reinforced by a consensus of agreement concerning the meaning of titles (mother, friend or lover). These consensus of agreements were suggested as being of great importance since they allowed people to weave a safety net for life. This, in turn, allows everyone to be what they are supposed to be and reinforce the location of the person in a concept of community or within a social network.

Chapter 3 developed this location into a notion of 'natives'. The native has his/her own customs, norms and language which bonds the sense of belonging and security. Natives share their beliefs in a public sense and this helps a group identity develop. Group identity fosters rituals of inclusion and exclusion which further bond the group. Group identity allows the natives to recognize that which is abnormal or the deviant. Acceptance to rejection, it is argued, normally occurs gradually but there can be catastrophic reaction of immediate rejection. In an attempt to signify the complexity of social life Chaos Theory was introduced to illustrate how each component of life touched and influenced the next. Just as Jimmy Stewart in *It's a Wonderful Life* could not be seen in isolation from his community, nor can a person's biology from his sociology and vice versa.

The concept of processing a deviant was explored and notions of exiles and refugees and this led into Chapter 4 which attempted to explore the terrain leading to the interior of the practitioner's world. Thus on to the inevitable illustration of the sick role.

The first four chapters have been designed to review the concept of societal living from a person and group of persons perspective. In short these chapters are essentially about people and how they live together. The last two chapters of Part One moved more into the macro-society by examining how impersonalized policies and concern for the majority often lost sight of the person. This has essentially influenced the first two chapters of Part Two, where caring has been explored from a majority view. At the end of the last chapter it was suggested that community care attempts to function on two levels, acute and chronic, and that there were two aspects, care in the community and care by the community. In addition the major theme of the text, so far, is that community care must, in both a theoretical and practical sense, be person-centred.

Care is a subjective notion. The act of caring is something personal, prompted by various motives and offered at various levels. Some people care for animals and are angered by any cruelty shown towards the smallest of beasts. Some even refuse to eat meat because of their concern for animals. Others are totally indifferent and some gain amusement through hunting and killing animals. If an animal-loving meat eater were to ask a fellow animal lover why they refuse to eat meat the chances are that he/she could not identify with the argument and vice versa, the vegetarian may not understand how an animal lover can eat meat. Getting to the root of why people care is futile since they are entrenched within the private self and, consequently, totally individual. In short there can be no universal meaning for caring. In this sense it is rather like pain, it can be experienced but observers can only ever gain a perception of another's experience (Buber, 1970). Hence, when we are interacting with people in the caring arena we have to accept that caring will range across a continuum of caring to non-caring. The amount of care a person can feel towards another will be the product of his/her experience through the atlas of existence. One has to be given care to develop an understanding of same. Care and attention are often blurred. Battered children, for example, often prefer natural parents who beat them than caring foster parents. The attention that natural parents give is seen as the norm. In some groups beating one's wife is seen as a display of affection (Skidmore, 1986). In other words, like other norms in society, one has to gather a sense of meaning from one's experience before the norm can be conformed to. If the messages are negative the chances are that a person will develop a negative view. Parents who beat their offspring tend to have been battered by their parents (Musa and Skidmore, 1991).

The notion of caring in a person's world will develop like all other norms. There will be a private and a public display. Should a person not give or receive care, then that is the norm in his/her world. No amount of professional skill can create caring artificially. If a person has constructed the reality of his/her world with an absence of caring then the likelihood is that they would not be interested in receiving care in the emotional sense.

At this stage, then, we have to distinguish from emotional and mechanical care. Mechanical care has been explored earlier in this section – it is the care offered through a sense of duty. Emotional care is the care delivered through affection for the person. Emotional care can also touch all the elements of a person's being: biological, sociological, psychological and political. Mechanical care is normally confined to the biological and attends to functional matters. Unfortunately there is a tendency to believe that mechanical care can be extended to the psychosocial aspects of life, the aspects of counselling alluded to in Part One (active listening and so on). The lobby against mechanical care has gained some support in the professional world. In the field of drug addiction some practitioners argue that it is 'caused' by social factors which cannot be altered so we should foster safe practice of drug taking. This is a natural outcome of enforcing a professional view on the world. The argument is that because a client does not respond to the professional's intervention then there is something wrong with the client and/or his/her world. It is rather like the attention given to the revolving door syndrome; the notion that because a client has not responded to several treatment regimens it is because they thrive on the attention. Rosenhan (1973) offers clues for this syndrome when he illustrated that professionals related to diagnoses and what they expected to see rather than what happened. The professional expects a client to respond and if he/she does not then the blame lies with the client. However, the behaviour that a professional brings to an encounter can advertise that he/she does not 'emotionally' care for the client. Repeated encounters will further confirm the prominence of mechanical care over emotional care.

We tend to allow certain people to be influential in our lives who we feel care 'emotionally' for us. During crises we are susceptible to outside influence and subsequently may transfer emotional connotations onto the therapist. When these are not reciprocated a sense of rejection is experienced. The previous chapters, in this part, stressed that giving a person responsibility in the process was crucial for success. Our previous experiences will have suggested to us that when others have taken over our lives it has been because of emotional care (parents for example). Therefore, when a person enters our lives, and we are in crisis, and that person takes control we can misunderstand the motives. Just as the professional may resort to the parental model as a guide for care the client may utilize the same in an attempt to understand the process. If a member of the opposite sex shows interest in a person it is almost always understood to be a display of attraction. Consequently there are dangers inherent in taking control of another's life. From each person's experience it is analogous with caring.

STARTING POINTS

The theme of this text has been that a person constructs his/her own meaning of community over time. They come to know that country very well and anchor their ideals to various landmarks in their country. Their community is a mixture of their public and private world. The closer to the centre of their community the more influential will be the private world, such as in the family. A suitable starting point, then, is to allow the client to guide the therapist through that community, rather than approaching the situation from the therapist being the guide. If the objective is to integrate the client into the community the therapist needs to know:

- the contours of the community prior to the condition;
- what has been disrupted and/or lost;
- what does the client wish to return to.

UNDERSTANDING THE ATLAS

Gaining a clear picture of how well located a person felt that they were within a community can offer useful information about how disconnected they now feel. The person who was most influential in the family and at work, and who had a wide circle of friends and colleagues will have had an extended community. These are often very difficult to repair. The person who was quite isolated and relied mainly on his immediate family for social interaction can be viewed as having a nuclear community. The nuclear community is much easier to repair. The nuclear community is founded on blood ties and affection whereas the extended community can be compared to the early industrial communities that required several links to bond people. The links that cement bonds are also important to identify. Sudden redundancy can be a major source of disconnectedness since it will often erode the bonds forged through work and those social bonds created outside work. In addition it will rob the person of their identity in several social circles. The image that we have of unemployment in the west is stigmatized to the extent that people now identify that which they are unemployed at. Revealing the previous job title suggests whether or not the unemployment is voluntary in some way. Certainly it helps to preserve the identity. Whereas almost anyone could claim to be an unemployed labourer a few questions would expose the falsely claimed unemployed biochemist.

The links a person feels that they have are the contours of their country/community. Where to go for certain favours or services, who can be relied on for support, who can be confided in and who will give advice; all these links are developed over time. Those people who are exiled from their community have lost all this and may never gain the level of access to others whereby they can be rebuilt. We take these links so much for granted that they become background expectancies. Background expectancies are so common place in our lives that we assume everyone has them without question. It is only when they disappear that we recognize their worth on a personal level. The dysfunctional person will start to question his/her connectedness and will recognize losses. Earlier in this text the suggestion was made that during divorce a person does not lose a partner but also part or whole of his/her community. People build contours based on mutual prediction. If prediction about a person, that is the ability to claim that a fellow native is like you, revolves around their married life being like yours, then an end to married life makes them different. The divorced person's friendship network is often disrupted until they become a couple again. These lost links can be explored and rated in terms of importance.

Naturally, some of these links will be severed for ever. No matter how skilled the professional is a divorced spouse cannot be forced into loving their 'ex'. Many relationships will disintegrate due to perceived betrayal, such as one partner's exposed infidelity. The nature of betrayal is that someone close to a person commits an act that would never have been predicted. The adage that the wife/husband is always the last to know is a contradiction in real terms. The wife/husband is best placed and knows their partner so well that they will recognize changes in behaviour and mood. However, like any deviance they will make attempts to normalize the changes, that is to explain them in some acceptable way. There will come a time, however, when the real reason has to be accepted and recognized (Davis, 1963). Once there is acceptance the whole basis of the relationship is catastrophically changed and every other predictable aspect of the relationship is brought into question. The act of betrayal declares that the other person is not like you, whereas the relationship was previously based on the premise that the person was. Skidmore (1986) described similar processes when friendships broke up. Skidmore (1986) argues that people built friendships on qualities that they had no right to expect. Unlike marriage, friends do not go through a ritual that contains vows and yet there appear to be unwritten rules that are agreed about the relationship.

A suitable starting point, then, for community care is to get to know the community in terms of a person's location, beliefs and values. Again this is a person-centred exercise. The only skill, at this stage, that the therapist needs to take to the encounter is that generated by a genuine interest in people, the skill of discovering their view of their country. If the therapist takes an instinctive dislike to the client, and this can happen, they should accept the feeling and refer the client to a colleague. Person-centred approaches require some form of positive regard for those you are attempting to help.

This starting point should inform that the whole process of community care is a partnership where the professional cannot claim total power. Hence the desires of the client have to be explored. In other words how much care does the client desire, from whom and at what level. There is little point in wasting resources and time with overkill if it simply alienates the client. Some people may gauge that attention from a professional in his/her community could be more harmful than helpful; this person may prefer non-intervention and that could be a reasonable request. The ultimate role of the professional is to facilitate the clients return to his/ her community. This could involve helping them to restructure or come to terms with some damaged aspects but the choice is the clients. If professionals are happy to discharge them in their own care then we have to accept their ability to make decisions governing their lives. The professional, then, is trying to sell the client a service by declaring in which areas he/she can be of assistance. If the client responds by insisting that he/she requires no help, then that choice has to be accepted if we are offering care in the community. The next step may be to negotiate care by the community.

Not to respect the wishes of the client in this direction is to remove their adult status. Insisting that a person receives community care is to invest the client with the status of an orphan. In other words to view them as a minor who needs either surrogate parents or the protection of an orphanage. We learn from experience that children lack the where-withal to care for themselves on various levels. They are unaware of many dangers, unable to feed themselves in a nutritious way and liable to be corrupted by others into a life of crime (the Fagin syndrome). Projecting this view onto clients is an extension of the parent-child model of care and carries the danger that we create a kingdom of orphans in the community. Placing a client in the orphan role can encourage the client to learn helplessness and fail to reconstruct or reclaim his/her community. Placing the person secondary to the condition can facilitate this. The person comes to be recognized by their label rather than their personhood. It may seem to be labouring a point but one must become aware that society has become increasingly secular. Bell (1956) suggested that the organic relationship had disappeared when the group tie of local community had shattered. It could be argued that the community has merely become more personalized but more important emotionally. The early industrial communities were much more formally structured by virtue of the many formalized links its members shared (marriage ties, kinship, workplace and social events). The community would have revolved around the workplace, linked its own timetable to that of the industry and shared group holidays. The move to the more privatized society (Tonnies, 1955) has allowed people to construct their own communities based on choice and self-projection. Consequently, when a person's community is threatened their very self-esteem is threatened.

It has been argued in Chapter 7 that the idealized organic community (gemeinschaft) is alive and well and living in the private world of the self. It is to be expected, then, that if a person's community starts to disintegrate they will experience a serious sense of loss because their very ideals are being challenged. The person's community is a projection of self. Since we feel that we know ourselves that sense of knowing is projected onto the community. To suddenly discover that we do not know it after all will plunge most people into a state of crisis. This is rather like being an orphan, having no links and feeling that one does not belong, and should the professional take a parental model to the encounter it would be easy for both parties to accept this role. Consequently it is important to explore, with a client, that which has survived. The nuclear family, for instance, may be something that can be identified and built upon. More important is to emphasize the survival of the person, since the person was previously the centre of their own world.

To facilitate a kingdom of orphans is to create institutionalization. The orphan is dependent upon the adult in most things. Similarly the client becomes a patient when dependent on the therapist and is more suited to institutional care. There is an argument that to allow clients to participate in professional decisions is a denial of professionalism. This is so if we are to accept professionalism as a process that gives a group a body of knowledge that they must control, and that that knowledge always benefits the wider society. With regard to many conditions that present in the hospital, patient involvement in decision making is inappropriate. The person in a state of collapse, for example, who needs emergency surgery. However, it has been argued that community care must function on an individual level, since a person constructs their own community. The person is allowing the professional access to that community and consequently must be party to any decision if it is to be adopted (Gellerman, 1972). In this instance allowing the client to participate in decision making is an enhancement of professionalism.

The professional who intervenes in community settings has a much more difficult task than those functioning in the institutional setting. Hence it will be much more difficult to let go of professional control. The institutional professional has the whole structure of the institution supporting him/her every minute of the working day. There are fellow professionals who can be consulted to support or modify decisions and the clients in this setting are much more passive. The community professional is very much more autonomous and will be required to make and defend decisions. In addition the client will be far less passive because they are not policed 24 hours a day. It takes a great deal of courage to allow participation in this setting. This is, one argues, why the professional has to be quite clear of the appropriate action: is it care in or by the community, is it a combination and can either be attained. This will depend upon the recognition of the acute or chronic nature of the condition and of a good knowledge of the person's community. If there are no community links and no desires for the same then care by the community, other than self-care, is unlikely.

Self-care is a viable alternative in the community setting. Care by the community does not need to involve other people if one accepts that the community is highly personalized. A person may wish to keep his condition secret in order to preserve his/her community which, after all, he/she knows better than anyone. Self-care does, however, rely on the transfer of a large amount of responsibility by the professional. Most diabetics engage in successful self-care and it has not negated the need for professionals. Society should not be misled into the belief that community care can only exist when others are involved. What society has accepted as community care in the past has often been the simple transfer of formal care to lay-carers. In this context community care means any care given in a person's concept of community. It refers to care that facilitates a person's location and connectedness with or without the assistance of others.

Most people indulge in some aspect of self-care throughout their lives. They utilize medications for the self-treatment of headaches, indigestion and other aches and pains. Many more people are taking an active part in preserving their health through exercise and sensible eating. Smoking cigarettes has declined on a national level in the UK, which could indicate that people are much more aware of health issues. The body is a complex organism and most people become very adept at caring for it. There are exceptions, there are those who abuse their bodies and seem determined to damage it in whatever way they can. There are those who do so less actively. The professionals are quite content to recognize these persons and refuse to give care unless they stop smoking or drinking or whatever. There is no equal recognition of those people who successfully look after their health. Nor is there a recognition that people may be quite effective self-care practitioners.

In short, then, intervention in the community is dependent upon the type of person and the construction of that community. It cannot be approached in a similar way to institutional care. Institutions are fairly static and respond to the group norm. Communities are varied and are the products of individual norms. The style of intervention required is totally different in that it has to be person-centred rather than condition specific; clients need to be involved in decisions, the goal being to hand responsibility over to the client in total. The programme of intervention can involve care in the community or care by the community or both. Care by the community may involve assistance from others or simple self-care. When others are involved, as foster parents or step-parents they will require professional support and education so as not to create dependence on the part of the client.

Care in the community is not a cheap option in terms of resources and care by the community is more than the simple transfer of responsibility. This text has explored the complexities of personhood and communities. If the person is to be safeguarded then each community care programme requires negotiation on the personal level. The dangers contained in ignoring the person is that we have the capabilities to create a kingdom of orphans who will make increasing demands on the welfare state to the detriment of its survival. The current example is of those orphans evicted from the mental hospitals who are now requiring special monitoring. The demands made by this group have been created by society. We should recognize this and accept this as a warning because the potential to create many more groups like this is enormous.

Care in and by the community is very much in favour and looks set to be the major form of health and welfare delivery by the year 2000. It has great potential with regard to safeguarding a state health care system and the dignity of the natives. At the same time, if we rush headlong into the community with an institutional mentality it can, and will, and does, cause great damage to the health and welfare services and the whole concept of community. Communities are important for the support of the person. We are all persons, if we are complicit in any process that damages the community we ultimately damage ourselves.

REFERENCES

Bell, D. (1956) The theory of mass society. *Commentary*, July.

Buber, M. (1970) *I and Thou*, T. and T. Clark, Edinburgh.

Davis, F. (1963) *Passage through Crisis*, Bobbs Merrill, Indianapolis.

Gellerman, S. (1972) *Behavioural Science in Management*, Penguin, Harmondsworth, Middlesex.

Marris, B. (1974) *Loss and Change*, Routledge and Kegan Paul, London.

Musa, A. and Skidmore, D. (1991) Child abuse and subsequent substance abuse. The Manchester Metropolitan University and Blackpool Health Authority, unpublished.

Nietzsche, F. (1977) *A Nietzsche Reader*, Penguin, Harmondsworth, Middlesex.

Rosenhan, D.L. (1973) On being sane in insane places. *Science*, **179**, 250–8.

Schutz, A. (1962) *The Problem with Social Reality: collected papers*, Martinus Nijhoff, The Hague.

Skidmore, D. (1986) The sociology of friendship. University of Keele, PhD Thesis.

Tonnies, F. (1955) *Community and Association*, Routledge and Kegan Paul, London.

CHAPTER 10

Adulthood/naturalization: empowerment and normalization

In this final chapter it is hoped that the whole concept of belonging will be drawn together and the similarities between geographical and kinship analogies will be identified (if they have not already been so). The final metaphor 'adulthood/naturalization' is adopted with one meaning to illustrate similarity.

The child seizes power and becomes an adult, it is never given. Skidmore (1993) argues that structured play prepares the child for an adult gender role and that within the framework of play the process of empowerment ensues. Chapter 3 discussed how different degrees of powerfulness could develop and one should be aware that not everyone desires to be a leader. Everyday power is concerned with managing one's life and knowledge of the rules of one's geography (Chapters 1 and 2) are crucial to the development of that power. Similarly the dominance of private self over public self will influence the amount of power seized (Goffman, 1969). Public life tends to contain black and white rules that we acknowledge, the colour is added by the private self. Rather like the movie *The Wizard of Oz*, real life commences in black and white film, the private life bursts into full colour.

Children develop into adults over a reasonably long period and have time to learn the rules, to enforce their private self onto the world, in short to become empowered. Children usually have the advantage of belonging to their society. Refugees have to become children again with no guarantee of being allowed to become adult. They may apply for naturalization but this is synonymous with adulthood.

Refugees and emigres can apply for nationality by way of a formal process. The principle underpinning naturalization is to provide a person with membership of a nation. There will, of course, always be the accent that betrays one's real origin or at least the notion that one does not truly belong. In essence giving the refugee a passport of the adopted country empowers that person, i.e. it authorizes his/her presence and, technically, enables free passage through the country and to other countries.

It is not, of course, as simple as the issuing of a passport. The west still has an appalling record of racism directed against its own nationals, i.e. those second and third generation children of immigrants. Indeed, the 1990s has witnessed a rise of nationalism in Western Europe that has led to structured attacks on ethnic minorities. Consequently we cannot accept legal residence and official papers as a token of membership. In Mills' (1970) terms racism has become a public issue. Mills distinguishes between private troubles and public issues. With regard to racism, Mills would argue that if a true minority (such as 1 in 100 000) were subjected to racial abuse then it is a private trouble, i.e. the person should be looked at for the solution, his personality for example. This is almost echoing Russell's argument (Chapter 5). However, when the statistics rise and a sizeable number of the community are victims then it becomes a public issue and we have to look beyond the individual to the very structure of society. Those requiring community care, the refugees of Chapter 3, appear to be viewed, politically at least, as private troubles and this brings into question the whole issue of community care generally and empowerment specifically. This will be further discussed below.

The introduction for this text and Chapter 1 outlined that the focus of this discourse was ideology. Joseph (1994) suggests that ideologies are used to justify the position of powerful people in society and that they may be distorted and not based on actual facts. Nietzsche (1977) offers similar arguments. Merton (1968) describes society by way of manifest and latent functions, or the ideology and the fact. Merton offers several examples such as education (manifest or ideology is to educate, latent or real is to produce a socially desirable type). The ideology underpinning naturalization is to offer membership, the latent function is often to produce victims and social isolation. Worsley (1987) claims that human behaviour is strongly influenced by the culture of the society in which they are natives. This could be extended, as Nietzsche (1977) suggests, in that the culture is the product of the ideals of the most powerful people. If so, then the only way to turn the ideology of naturalization into a reality would be to change the culture and wait. The wait would be necessary for the owners of the old belief systems to die out. Worsley's (1987) view of culture is central to the understanding of ideology. He views culture as a collection of norms and values held by society (Chapter 2). The norms, as has been argued above, form the framework by which we judge normality. For a person to belong to a group he has to be predictable; to be predictable he has to be like the rest; to be like the rest he has to mirror the norms of the group which extends to appearance, accent and traditional knowledge. In short he must not be walking the tightrope. Many immigrants sound different and look different, this makes them unpredictable. Joseph (1994) suggests that immigrants can change their beliefs and behaviour (and become members) whilst others in the same group do not change and remain in the 'ghetto'. One could take issue with Joseph on two points:

1. Membership is greater than beliefs and behaviour. A person can do little about his appearance or others knowledge of his background.
2. People can be shunted into ghettos by housing policies and non-acceptance by the natives.

Membership or nativeness is a combination of things that contributes to the symbol of belonging. It has been argued, above, that we define first and then see (Lippman, 1922). Bergson (1918) states that true perception, that is seeing things for the first time without ascribing use and meaning, is only possible in theory whilst ever we have knowledge of the past. The symbol of belonging is very much dependent on how others see us. When we view another person we immediately take in a wealth of information: history, location, appearance, status. The other person's response to us informs of whether or not they share the same beliefs and knowledge.

We tend to know whether or not a person shares a similar **history** by having knowledge of their place of birth, schooling, occupation and family. This aspect of connectedness has been discussed in Chapter 2. Shared history contributes to our understanding of a person's social **location**, i.e. where he/she is placed in terms of a relationship with self: friend or relative. An understanding of a person's history and location helps define his/her **status** in the society. The person's **appearance**, i.e. behaviour, looks and language, reinforces views on whether or not that person belongs and stereotyping may cause the observer not to interact and test out beliefs and knowledge.

Consequently a great deal is assumed about a person from that which we feel they project symbolically (Carlyle, 1908).

Consequently, the ideology of equality is nothing more than rhetoric whenever the beliefs of the dominant take precedence over the weak. Fortunately many minority groups have effective advocates who have done much to change policy and make society treat some groups with more dignity.

EMPOWERMENT – ENFORCED

The statement that power is seized and never given was made at the beginning of this chapter. Empowerment in the therapeutic sense appears to favour giving, not facilitating taking. In some senses it is even enforced, an issue discussed later. It has been stated, above, that empowerment is understood to mean: to authorize or enable. In one sense it is about enabling a person to make informed choices, in another it gives a person the authority to act on that choice. Embodied in the ideology of community care is the notion of empowerment. The very act of placing a person in a community makes a statement about that person having responsibility. There is also an assumption that the person desires to be empowered. Empowerment is virtually impossible without status.

If we consider the care of the long term mentally ill, one could argue that they have always belonged to an underclass (Joseph, 1994). However, when they were inmates of the institution they could, at least, negotiate status within the 'underclass society'. Removing them, in small numbers, to different parts of a 'community' has, in effect, deconstructed their society and to a large extent disempowered them. It should be remembered that some people are quite happy being looked after and subsequently disempowered (Chapter 4). Skidmore (1979) reported that a significant number of people gained a sense of security from investing total faith in the medical arena and passively following instruction. The long term mentally ill have been schooled in a culture that places them in an underclass where they lived their lives for the good of the institution (Goffman, 1961; Illich, 1976). To a large degree they came to terms with that and developed a concept of 'nativeness', where they belonged to a culture. Suddenly they are removed from their culture and placed on a tightrope in a strange culture where they are expected to become empowered with little knowledge of the culture. Similarly they are expected to be 'normalized'. Their removal was brought about with uninformed consent which contradicts the concept of empowerment. In the same vein we have discussed how the insulin-dependent diabetic can be empowered but the phenothiazine-'dependent' person is discouraged from empowerment. This is another example of the rhetoric of community care. Community care assumes that the person has and desires power. The person who has suffered long term mental illness is in a similar status position to the child. The child has to undertake established rituals before they are allowed to seize power. The discharged long term mentally ill has no such rituals and, metaphorically, is destined to be a child forever.

EMPOWERMENT – DESIRED

It has been suggested in this text that many disabled people wish to be enabled. Those who suddenly have a physical disability through trauma, for example, may wish to seize control of their lives again. The process of rehabilitation is essentially about empowerment. However, part of that process must involve needs assessment. The disabled person may only be in a position to live a near normal life with the investment of extra resources. The analogy is that of the rich man: a rich man can achieve most of the things he desires by virtue of his wealth; the poor man makes do with his lot. The disabled are the poor of the welfare state. Political empowerment does not necessarily support individual empowerment. Again, the notion of community care requires a true sharing of power between clients and their carers (Sines, 1993). This is a process that neither clients nor carers are schooled in. Empowering one requires the disempowerment of the other. Sines (1993) argues that some professionals believe that their own interests are of primary importance. Unfortunately this is a human failing and we often assume that professionals can rise above the usual human emotions.

The physically disabled can often be identified by simple observation and the observer will immediately ascribe meaning to that which is seen. Under such circumstances it is difficult to ascribe the same behaviours as a 'native' because we imagine ourselves in that position and that which we would lose. Unfortunately rehabilitation tends to be concentrated on the disability rather than holistically, i.e. how to manage with one hand and come to terms with an altered body image. Although these issues are important they do not address the needs of the total person and rarely touch on the necessary social skills now required (Chapter 5) (Hodges, 1991). To facilitate the desired empowerment of a client means a full assessment of needs and the wherewithal to provide the necessary resources. It has been discussed throughout this text that such an option is not practical under the present and future economic climate.

The Health Care system in Finland offers an admirable service to the elderly and the disabled, but it is now suffering because of the recession (Skidmore, 1993). The elderly with Alzhiemer's disease are cared for in homes where they have their own rooms. Couples are also catered for and the carers make much use of family objects, photographs, favourite chairs and reminiscence. There is very minimal use of drugs and a very relaxed and happy atmosphere can be witnessed. Unfortunately families are now having to contribute far more and many such homes are being privatized and community care is being promoted by central government. The manifest function of community care is to provide a better quality of life. The latent function is to shift the responsibility for care provision. The process of empowerment by central government is linked to economy rather than needs. Those persons desiring empowerment may be better served by adjustment therapy unless the necessary resources can be found.

Empowerment has occurred on a professional level by creating the purchaser-provider system. The actual focus of health care has effectively been changed from one of caring to that of working within a budget (Chapter 5). The outcome of such a change is to dismantle the welfare state where treatment is free regardless of the cost. The reality is that the ethos of political empowerment (transferring responsibility) is reinforced by the professional carers. Primary care has been received with enthusiasm by professionals since its proposed expansion by Griffiths (1988). Griffiths proposed that local needs should be assessed by local social service authorities and then forward planning could occur that would meet those needs. The local authorities then suffered a change in funding which meant that many local services had to be axed (such as meals on wheels). Joseph (1994) argues that those who really lose out by the failure to meet needs are disabled people, former inpatients who are now homeless and carers. Primary care is based on the care of the individual in the community; when the quality of care is removed the reality is that primary care has permitted the move to care based on individualism and finance: care based on costs and the ability to pay (Chapter 5).

In short, then, the current provision of community care is incongruent with the notion of empowerment. However, human beings are innovative and are able to seize power by various means and that can create problems for community carers. Black *et al.* (1984) suggest that some people use their condition to gain power because that is all they have left. A person may emphasize their disability in order to gain advantage. This can have the effect of reinforcing the stereotyped image of the disabled and push them further into that role. Certainly the current policy for the mentally ill is creating negative empowerment; that is using a condition to impinge on the lives of others. Negative empowerment has led to the policy changes described in Chapter 5 which will, in turn, negate any attempts to empower positively. This process is a more refined form of institutionalization. Within the institution (prisons for example) inmates develop a type of negative culture: status through violence or wealth by way of tobacco; similarly a negative culture may develop at a smaller level in the 'community'. In Chapter 3 the concept of 'social death' was introduced. Social death is a way of categorizing a person's existence when they become totally ineffective within their immediate culture. A biological metaphor would be the person without any of the senses (sensory deprivation). The western culture stimulates a person to fight against social death and in an attempt to gain resurrection strategies are devised that will cause acknowledgement by the outside world. Hence a continuum of empowerment could be suggested:

positive	social	negative
empowerment	death	.... empowerment

In Chapter 3 the notion of catastrophic action was discussed. The move from positive to negative empowerment may be a gradual process over many years or it may catastrophically plunge from positive to negative. It may even be a combination of the two processes and a catastrophic swing may occur at any point on the continuum.

Empowerment of any kind is strongly linked to independence and that is a desire of most people: the choice of when one goes to bed or eats or goes for a walk. Johnstone (1993) argues that discharged schizophrenics prefer to stay out of hospital because in the hospital they lack independence. It is every person's right to make informed decisions about their life. To make decisions knowledge is required. Many of the long term mentally ill were not provided with realistic information prior to discharge. Consequently when they discover that they are in an environment where they are isolated and threatened with social death they are likely to seize negative empowerment. In the more dramatic cases the media seize onto the story and add to the stigmatization of the group, creating a medium for even greater social death. The recent (1993) coverage of the Rollins case (described as a schizophrenic who stabbed his father to death) is just one more nail into the coffin which will disempower the disabled. Johnstone (1993) quite rightly comments that most people who stab another are not psychotic. However, the sensational reports on such cases create a barrier between these groups and the general public. The isolated person is unable to utilize the conservative impulse (Chapter 1) since he cannot use the reactions of those around him in the present to decide future actions. He, in fact, enters a process of social anomie or normlessness which in turn will lead to social death. This will steer the person to mix with similar groups in the community, the process of secondary normalization discussed in Chapter 3. Such a group will be supportive in a negative way, in that it encourages the very behaviour that alienates the rest of the public. If social skills are identified as a major necessity for social integration then these are central to the process of empowerment. All the world is a stage, to paraphrase Shakespeare, but you have to know how to act and which play is now showing. The focus for community preparation is on alleviating the symptoms and assuming that everything else will come right.

Earlier in this chapter it was suggested that it takes years to become an adult, but one can become a child again overnight. Once a child all power is removed except that which can be claimed through negative means. When a child screams he quickly learns that it brings attention with it. The deviant is merely utilizing that learning process. What the rest of us have to come to terms with is the fact that few other options are left open to these people. A political voice has to be built up through sympathetic groups and often this takes years (from child to adult again); SANE and MIND are examples of such groups. Consequently when considering the notions of empowerment, normalization and rehabilitation, they have to be considered alongside choice. Hugman (1992) argues that the exercise of choice is more than acquiring the necessary social skills, it extends to the range of possibilities that are available in the shape of services and accommodation. Empowerment is concerned with giving the client equal power and a choice in the style of intervention. Clough (1982) argues that participation should be a right for service users and Brandon (1981) suggests that psychiatric services should be based on the experiences of service users. Both lines of argument have validity if service provision were to start from year zero, i.e. without bringing a history with it. However, because the past of a thing is always viewed alongside its present (Chapter 1), totally changing direction in the future is unlikely. Hugman (1992) suggests that helping people to exercise choice is a complex practice issue and may be limited by the actual range of options which exist for a person.

It has been discussed in Chapters 1, 2 and 4 that people develop different levels of power through life due to the interrelationship of their biological, sociological and psychological components. Some will be born disadvantaged, due to a deformity for example, but will not necessarily display political weakness unless their sociology and psychology push them in that direction. Of course some people gain comfort in certain situations by allowing others to take control. Caplan (1964) suggests that during crises people are much more vulnerable to outside influence and much more likely to allow others to take control of their lives. Empowerment, then, is a two-way process. The client has to desire power and the therapist/carer must wish to hand it over. Given that both parties will carry a historical view about each other and 'power', this does indeed become problematical. Buckley (1968) argues that society is a complex adaptive system. The interchanges between the components can change significantly and this may result in changes in the nature of the components themselves with consequences for the system as a whole. This was the process suggested in Chapter 3, with the adaptation of Hodges' Health Career Model, on an individual level. To modify Buckley's argument the interchanges within society can change the nature of the inhabitants with consequences for the whole of society. We are currently witnessing a deconstruction of the welfare state and hear warnings that it is happening elsewhere (Pylkkanen, 1993). Manifestly this is to offer a better quality of care to the client by empowering them, normalizing them or rehabilitating them. The act of empowering is seen as a simple act, divorced from the resource issue, financial aspects and personal preference. Enforcing a person to take responsibility is as negative as neglect. Topliss (1982) suggests that normalization is another form of neglect. In the context that they are being used we could add empowerment and rehabilitation to the acts of neglect.

Therapists and carers have to grasp the nettle of advocacy and make sure that it is the client's will that is being considered and not the party-line. The latter is much easier because we do not have to consider important components such as available resources, we can transfer that responsibility. The former is closer to the complex issues debated by Hugman (1992) and would require a significant amount of resources to implement. Care in the community is not a cheap option if carried out effectively. Transferring responsibility of care to clients and their families is. The consequences of following the party-line have been discussed in Chapter 5, empowering the client will do little to save the welfare state.

REFERENCES

Bergson, H. (1918) *The Philosophy of Change*, T.C. & E.C. Jack, London.

Black, N., Boswell, D., Gray, A. *et al.* (1984) *Health and Disease*, The Open University Press, Milton Keynes.

Brandon, D. (1981) *Voices of Experience: consumers perspectives of psychiatric treatment*, MIND, London.

Buckley, W. (1968) Society as a Complex Adaptive System, in *Modern Systems Research for the Behavioural Sciences* (ed. W. Buckley), Aldine, Chicago.

Caplan, G. (1964) *Principles of Preventative Psychiatry*, Tavistock, London.

Carlyle, T. (1908) *Sartor Resartus*, Dent, London.

Clough, R. (1982) *Residential Work*, Macmillan, London.

Goffman, E. (1961) *Asylums*, Penguin, Harmondsworth, Middlesex.

Goffman, E. (1969) *The Presentation of Self in Everyday Life*, Penguin, Harmondsworth, Middlesex.

Griffiths, R. (1988) *Community Care: agenda for action*, HMSO, London.

Hodges, B.E. (1991) Participant observations of rehabilitation. The Manchester Metropolitan University, unpublished.

Hugman, R. (1992) Rehabilitation and community support. *Applied Community Studies Journal*, **1**(2).

Illich, I. (1976) *Limits to Medicine*, Penguin, Harmondsworth, Middlesex.

Johnstone, E. (1993) Bringing psychotics to the fold. *THES*, 1098, 19 November.

Joseph, M. (1994) *A Sociology for Nursing and Health Care*, Polity Press, Cambridge.

Lippman, W. (1922) *Public Opinion*, Macmillan, London.

Merton, W. (1968) *Social Theory and Social Structure*, Free Press, New York.

Mills, C.W. (1970) *The Sociological Imagination*, Penguin, Harmondsworth, Middlesex.

Nietzsche, F. (1977) *A Nietzsche Reader*, Penguin, Harmondsworth, Middlesex.

Pylkkanen, K. (1993) We must act as the conscience of our society. *Newsletter of the Finnish Association for Mental Health*, 1.

Sines, D. (1993) Balance of power. *Nursing Times*, **89**(46), 52–5.

Skidmore, D. (1979) Anxiety in Medical Arenas. Cranfield Institute of Technology, MSc Dissertation.

Skidmore, D. (1993) *Report on Study Tour of Finland*, The Manchester Metropolitan University.

Topliss, E. (1982) *Social Responses to Handicap*, Longman, London.

Worsley, P. (1987) *The New Introductory Sociology*, Macmillan, London.

Author index

Subject index

Page numbers appearing in bold refer to figures.